Breast Care Options

Breast Care Options

A Cancer Specialist Discusses
Breast Care Options,
Risk Factors, and How to
Cope with Breast Cancer

Paul Kuehn, M.D.

Newmark Publishing Company

Published by Newmark Publishing Company
South Windsor, CT 06074
(203) 282-7265

Designed by Irving Perkins Associates
Typeset by NK Graphics
Printed and Bound by The Book Press
Manufactured in the United States of America

10 9 8 7 6 5 4 3 2 1

Library of Congress Cataloging in Publication Data

Kuehn, Paul
Breast Care Options
1. Risk Factors   2. Limited Surgery vs. Mastectomy   3. Stress, Diet

86-61100

ISBN 0-938539-00-0

First Edition

Contents

Appendix

Acknowledgments

This book is written as a guide for women with breast problems. A great deal of the information presented here has either not been published or is available only in medical journals which are not readily accessible to the public. Those publications that were invaluable throughout the writing of this book are numbered and included in a reference section at the end, as are the names and affiliations of medical specialists cited in the various chapters.

The health organizations mentioned in the book are included in the Appendix. Although several authorities read and criticized chapters related to their fields of expertise for accuracy, the viewpoints taken in advocacy or opposition are entirely my own.

I wish to thank my wife, Barbara, for her help with the statistical analysis of the questionnaire and my daughter, Carolyn, for the initial editing and critique of the book. I appreciate the many long hours they spent working with me.

To my secretary and typist, Judy Sharp, for her patience, skill and devoted effort to this book, I extend my deepest gratitude.

Thanks also to the many internationally known clinicians, researchers, and authorities whose scientific studies and observations have made this book possible.

Finally, to my patients, who unselfishly shared their personal and sometimes painful experiences with me, my debt is deep. It is they who have taught me about breast cancer, human nature and compassion and have helped make the publication of this book possible.

Introduction

This book is written for the woman who develops a lump in her breast which may be cancer and wishes to be fully informed about her breast care options.

As recently as ten years ago, when a woman had breast cancer it was considered a deep, dark secret. The very word caused fear among friends and relatives of victims as well as among victims themselves.

The unreasoning fear began to dissipate after two well known women—Betty Ford and Happy Rockefeller—announced that they had undergone mastectomies because of breast cancer. This openness has been immensely beneficial. After all, how can we deal with a problem unless we can discuss it and with cancer, there is much to discuss.

For example; recent advances in detection using new sophisticated imaging devices such as mammography, makes it possible to take a picture of the breast and spot many breast cancers when you can't even feel them. The cure rate for such minimal cancers is virtually one hundred percent. Some breast cancers can now be detected early enough to permit limited surgery instead of breast removal, and for those women who have a more advanced breast cancer and must undergo a mastectomy, the art of breast reconstruction has progressed immensely with markedly improved techniques and results.

In the past, cancer has been made to look fearsome, inexplicable, or a matter of chance. It is not. Staying healthy is frequently a matter of *choice*. When you read the stories in this book of women who survived cancer, you will see that their survival was a matter of faith; in themselves, their physicians, and treatments that helped them to overcome the disease. In still other cases, their faith took the form of an over-powering will to survive, a refusal to admit even the possibility of defeat.

Not all cancer is preventable. But *all* cancers respond better to treatment when detected in the early stages. Cancer seems to have many causes. A normal cell may be transformed into a malignant one as a result of viruses, radiation and chemicals such as food additives. Hormones, drugs, certain foods, even stress may enhance your chances of developing breast cancer. Predisposition to cancer may also be inherited. All of these factors are discussed in this book, using available research and the comments of patients who were sent an extensive questionnaire.

An attempt is also made to simplify some of the arguments and controversies concerning the treatment of breast cancer based upon my own experience with over four thousand women patients with breast disease. You will find in reading this book that there are still many controversies in how breast cancer should be treated. I have tried to discuss all the important breast care options that a woman should know about so that she may be better informed.

It is every woman's right—and responsibility—to learn the facts. This book can help. Through my own work with women it became clear to me that those who were able to conquer cancer had a formula for survival. They were determined to be victors, not victims. This book then is a logical extension of their medical education—and of mine. When women can begin talking about cancer as a fact of life without excessive fear, they can face it, fight it, and win.

PAUL KUEHN, M.D.

1

The Disease Women Fear Most

Breast cancer exists in all parts of the world and is seen more often in western civilizations.

The disease is apparently influenced by many factors—heredity, childbearing, possible viruses and, according to some authorities, a diet high in fats. None of the suspected causes, however, explain why in the United States, breast cancer is on the increase.

In the United States, more than 120,000 breast cancers are discovered each year according to statistics compiled by the National Cancer Institute. Almost one-half of these, when first found, show evidence of spread outside the local area of the breast and a significant number have spread throughout the body.[1,2] This suggests that something is wrong in our methods of detection and prevention.

Since breast cancer is on the increase, it is important that all women know the specific warning signs so they may be better able to detect any abnormality in their breasts.

Certain women are at greater risk to get breast cancer and an attempt should be made to identify these women so they may be watched more closely.

In my study of breast tumor patients (more than four thousand women), office charts were reviewed and all patients were asked to respond to a questionnaire. Over ninety percent responded and that data has been

1

used to substantiate previous studies and research concerning specific risk factors in breast cancer. It has also been helpful in setting up criteria for the evaluation and treatment of patients.

IMPORTANT RISK FACTORS

There has been considerable controversy as to whether breast cancer originates from a single cell that goes haywire and then multplies, invades tissue, and spreads to vital organs, or is a systemic disease from its onset.

Before consulting the chart of risk factors (Figure 1), you should know that: You have a *decreased* risk of breast cancer if you have no family history of breast disease, gave birth before age thirty, and had early menopause.

Heredity For families where breast cancer strikes several members, questions about heredity become inevitable. In my practice, seven percent of patients with breast cancer had mothers with the disease and twenty-one percent had aunts, grandmothers or sisters with breast cancer.

Heredity and genetic factors have been studied before. Numerous researchers, including Dr. Abraham M. Lilienfeld[3] and Dr. Madge T. Macklin,[4] showed that there is a marked increase when female relatives have breast cancer, including cousins, aunts and grandmothers. My own review of breast cancer patients substantiates these previous studies.

Age Ninety percent of the breast cancers that occurred in my practice had their onset after age thirty-eight. Ten percent developed in the younger age group. The youngest patient I treated was twenty-four and the oldest was ninety.

More than half of the breast cancers presented between the age of thirty-eight and fifty-four. The majority of the patients developed breast cancer at the menopause or later.

This makes monthly self-examination and annual checkups a lifetime must. It also suggests that the hormonal changes which occur at menopause play an important part in the etiology of breast cancer.

Children Another important factor in breast cancer is whether the patient has had children and how many. This is the subject of some

Figure 1
RISK FACTORS FOR BREAST CANCER

RISK FACTORS	Breast Cancer Incidence*		

Age

10%	50%	40%

Menopause

Years   38   54   90

90% after 38 yrs. of age

Heredity	Family history of breast cancer
	Family history other types cancer

Race	Higher incidence among white women--world wide

Children	Nulliparous (no children)
	Late birth of first child

Menopause	Women who continue menstruating late in life-- over 50 yrs.

Weight	Overweight

Diet	High triglyceride diet (high in fat, low in fiber)
	High beef intake.*

Hormones	Early start of menstruating (before 12 yrs.)
	? Birth control pill
	? Estrogen therapy

Thyroid Problems	Usually hypothyroid.
	? Stress

Socioeconomic status	Affluent, high income (may be related to diet)

Stress	? personality, depression

Drugs	Women exposed to DES

*Author's statistics

debate, but there is little question that nulliparous women—those who have no children—are high-risk candidates. It has also been widely accepted that bearing the first child at an early age confers some protection, for reasons as yet unknown. In one study of Catholic nuns, Dr. J.F. Fraumeni[5] found that the incidence of breast cancer was dramatically higher than the general female population. Another researcher[6] has shown that unmarried women have a higher risk of malignant tumors affecting the breast and reproductive organs.

Women who continue to menstruate late in life also have a definite increased risk for breast cancer. For this reason, I carefully watch childless women and those who are still menstruating after age fifty and examine them more often. This includes examination of the uterus and ovaries as well as the breasts.

Race Not only does breast cancer seem to be geographical, it has a higher incidence among white women than women of other races—a pattern that seems to prevail all over the world.

According to epidemiologists (those who study epidemic diseases including cancer in relation to environment and ways of life), the person most likely to develop breast cancer is a white woman of northern European descent who is overweight, had a relative with cancer, began menstruating early, and had a first child after she was thirty-five years old.

Overweight and Diet Being overweight is another factor that increases the risk of developing a malignant tumor. Not only that, excess weight can also make it more difficult to find one that is already there. When my patients were asked to rate themselves as to whether they felt they were average, below average, or overweight before they developed breast cancer, half said they were overweight and very few said they were underweight.

When asked which specific foods they liked to eat frequently, forty-five percent named steak and hamburgers. Cheese, butter, eggs, ice cream and fried foods were also high on the list. All of which is further evidence that a diet high in fat and low in fiber is associated with a tendency to develop breast cancer. This is discussed in more detail in Chapter 10—Cancer and the Foods You Eat.

Hormones and Menopause Women who begin menstruating at an earlier age (in the United States, before twelve) are more likely to develop breast cancer. On the other hand, if a woman has her ovaries removed before she is thirty-five, or has a natural menopause at an early age, her chances of developing breast cancer drop considerably.

The female sex hormone, estrogen, has long been known to produce breast cancer in animal experiments and estrogens have also been shown to cause pre-cancerous changes in breast tissue in humans. The lining of the ductal system of the breast can be stimulated by hormones (estrogens) to cause a condition (hyperplasia) that is known to progress on to breast cancer.

Estrogens are used in oral contraceptives and are often used in the treatment of hot flashes at the menopause. Some physicians feel that estrogens help prevent the bone crippling disease called osteoporosis. Research has shown that women who have never taken oral contraceptives have fewer malignant tumors than those who do.

When asked whether they took oral contraceptives or not, fifteen percent of my patients who developed breast cancer said they had. As to whether oral contraceptives actually cause cancer in humans there is no proof at the present time. Only further study will show if they produce carcinogenic effects on the breast, and in what numbers.

Fortunately, the oral contraceptives now in use have much lower estrogen content than when they were first introduced over thirty years ago and the risk factor may be decreased.

Many women have their uterus and ovaries removed at an earlier age than the menopause. Since the ovaries are the major source of estrogens, replacement therapy has to be given. Seventeen percent of the breast cancer patients that I treated had a total hysterectomy (uterus) and bilateral oophorectomy (ovaries). The estrogen replacement therapy was variable in dosage but all received estrogens. It is obvious that when the ovaries are removed and replacement estrogen therapy is given, a woman can still get breast cancer and no protective effect of the removal of the ovaries occurs.

If you need replacement estrogen therapy, the minimum estrogen dose should be used and carefully adjusted by your physician.

More information on hormones and breast cancer can be found in Chapter 5 and 6, which discuss pregnancy and the female reproductive system.

Thyroid Researchers[7,8,9] have been working for years on the relationship between thyroid disease and breast cancer, and they are certain there is a connection that involves iodine deficiency. However, it is difficult to establish the amount of risk involved. Of my breast cancer patients, twenty percent had a history of thyroid problems and seven percent had been operated on for thyroid disease. As to how the thyroid gland is involved in breast cancer, is not clear at the present time. The thyroid gland plays a role in maintaining a stable metabolism in the human body and also plays a role in stress and the immune system (Chapter 11).

Environment Only within the past few years has much attention been paid to the possible role of the environment in relation to breast cancer. Today, when we have more and more potentially harmful substances all around us, the "why" of breast cancer has become increasingly significant.

For example, women who live in cities have a higher incidence of breast cancer than those in rural areas. Those with higher income and social status are at greater risk[10]—presumably because they can afford the foods that make up a diet rich in fat and chemical additives.

Stress and Smoking The relationship of stress and women's status in society might be called the social psychology of cancer. There is no longer any doubt that stress has a marked effect on the body's functions. This is discussed in detail in Chapter 11, which concerns the body's immune system and stress, and in Appendix D.

As to how the physician should evaluate stress as a risk factor in breast cancer, a few points can be made here: There is growing evidence that resistance to cancer is immunologic in nature, and that several stress factors are exhibited in many patients with cancer. They are: depression prior to cancer development, relative inability to express hostile feelings, unresolved tension concerning a familial figure, and sexual problems.

Among my breast cancer patients, nearly forty percent said that they were under severe stress before the breast cancer was discovered. By contrast, among noncancerous control patients, a similar personality pattern involving stress was found in only ten percent.

Women who smoke may not develop breast cancer, but they are at higher risk of lung cancer, stomach ulcers, and heart disease. The lung is also a common site of spread of breast cancer, and the damaging effects of smoking do not ease the role of the physician. If my patient has breast cancer and smokes, she is vigorously advised to quit. Any way is okay—cold turkey, clinics, hypnosis—just as long as she quits. Not only does this make my job easier, but it makes the patient feel better and they all seem to do better.

Previous breast lumps and surgical biopsy as a risk factor Before the development of newer diagnostic aids to help the surgeon determine which patients needed to be biopsied for possible breast cancer, many women in the 1960's and early 1970's had biopsies whenever they developed a new lump in their breast. The most common cause for biopsy was fibrocystic disease and there were many surgeons who felt that fibrocystic disease was a precancerous condition.

Caffeine, chocolate, tea, and certain foods have been suggested as causative factors in fibrocystic disease. The biopsy of these numerous patients with fibrocystic disease has allowed a study of many patients that have been watched for many years since the tissue has been analyzed. I reviewed all of my patients that were biopsied and had a tissue diagnosis of fibrocystic disease (more than 500 cases). Less than one percent of these patients have gone on to develop cancer of the breast, suggesting that fibrocystic disease is not a pre-cancerous condition.

SUMMARY

In considering risk factors, there is an important difference to remember. They may not be actual cause and effect. For example, living in a city may be coincidental, not contributory—no one knows, and women must respect the high-risk factors that have been identified. She should also be sure her physician is aware of her risk status. As a woman approaches the menopause her risk increases and then continues for the rest of her life. Each woman is a separate individual and her risk factors can be quite variable.

2

Breast Self-Examination

Breast self-examination can save your life. Detecting breast cancer early, when the disease is in a more curable stage allows many new options in treatment and increases the chance of success and cure. Women know they *should* examine their breasts, but most don't.

A study has shown that only thirty-five percent of American women interviewed were examining their own breasts on a monthly basis.[11]

Secondly, breast self-examination results in earlier diagnosis. Evidence for this is the fact that as self-examinations are taught to women in screening programs, more of these women will detect their own cancers.[12]

Why don't more women examine their breasts? One problem is that few women have been taught to understand just what they're feeling. Breasts are naturally somewhat lumpy: They contain glandular tissue, fat, connective tissue, and lie over bone. They aren't sure about what's normal because they have never had a doctor or nurse take their hand, put it over their breast and say, "Feel this—this is your rib, this is a gland, this is breast tissue."

A number of women also are apprehensive and afraid to do breast self-examination. They should ask their doctor or nurse to do it for them, or at least show them how. (See Figure 2) This will allay most fears, especially if they are told that most lumps are benign. An ob-

Figure 2
BREAST SELF-EXAMINATION (BSE)

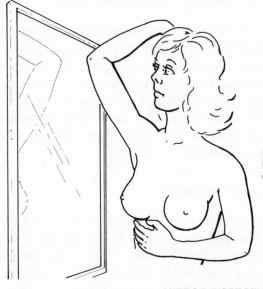

Look for skin
indentation, size
change and asymetry.

MIRROR INSPECTION

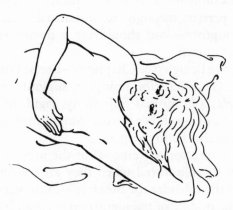

Feel for lumps completely
around the breast. Check
armpit. Press firmly, then gently.

LYING DOWN--PALPATING BREASTS

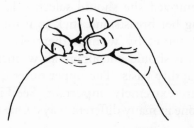

Squeeze nipple for
discharge: ? Bloody.
? Ulceration or other
abnormalities.

NIPPLE INSPECTION

stetrician is a good choice for women to consult and was the doctor most often consulted in my study of breast cancer patients (twelve percent).

In addition, many hospitals give individual instruction in breast self-examination (BSE) as part of their screening and diagnostic services. The American Cancer Society's *Teach-In* program gives free group instruction through local chapters. The instruction is given in the American Cancer Society booklet, available from local chapters. However, most instructions, excellent as they are, may omit some symptoms simply for lack of space in a small booklet. If you have any questions, you should consult with your doctor.

ONCE A MONTH, EVERY MONTH

Women twenty years of age or older should examine their breasts once a month, every month. The best time to do it is right after your menstrual period. The emphasis should be on familiarizing yourself with the way your breasts normally feel so you'll notice any change.

If you are in the age group that has annual mammograms, you should still do monthly breast self-examinations. If you do notice a change, especially in one breast that persists through the menstrual cycle—a lump, swelling, or other symptom—you should see a doctor right away. Never try to diagnose yourself.

Fortunately, most lumps prove benign (see Chapter 4—Breast Lumps That Are Not Cancer). Some characteristics, however, suggest cancer more than others. For example, a lump that feels stony, rigid, or has uneven edges should make a woman call her doctor. Skin dimpling or inversion of the nipples should also be investigated.

Women who have had a hysterectomy (removal of the uterus) but whose ovaries are intact may be able to tell when they are ovulating and should mark that date on the calendar for breast self-examination. Ovulation usually occurs in the middle of the menstrual cycle and may be accompanied by pain or discomfort in the lower abdomen. If a woman has had her ovaries removed she should select a day of the month at random for examining her breasts and stick to it for life.

Most breast cancers are still found by women themselves (about eighty percent in my study). This should encourage all women to do breast self-examination on a monthly basis. The upper outer quadrant of the breast and armpit area are extremely important. See Figure 3. Breast self-examination can be done in many different ways. One method may be better than another for each individual. The importance of BSE increases as the woman gets older. The monthly exam teaches the woman where small abnormalities are present and if a lump occurs, she can recognize it in the breast. There are many ways to do this examination. The method the patient feels most comfortable with is the one that she should use.

HOW YOU SHOULD DO IT

There are several ways to examine your breasts, but this three-stage procedure is the one found most effective: mirror inspection, breast palpation, and soaping the breasts. What is the reason for this? No *single* method of breast examination is best for finding the many symptoms of breast cancer, any of which call for a visit to the doctor.

Figure 3
LOCATION OF MOST BREAST CANCER LUMPS

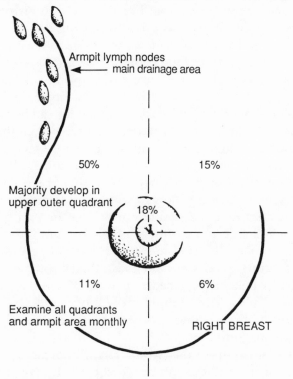

Statistics Source: National Cancer Institute

Mirror Inspection Stand in front of a large mirror and examine your breasts—first with your arms hanging at your sides, then with your hands pressing inward and down on your hips (to contract the pectoral muscles). Next press your palms together at heart level and, finally, clasp your hands behind your head. What you should be looking for:

1. *Skin dimpling* If the previously round contour of the breast becomes concave at any point, developing a dimple, the depression may indicate the pull of a tumor.
2. *Inversion of the nipple* A nipple that changes direction—pointing inward instead of projecting, or markedly shifting its angle— may signal an embedded tumor. It can also be the normal result of previous surgery, fibrocystic disease or calcium deposits.
3. *Nipple sore or irritation* One type of breast cancer is associated with nipple changes, Paget's Disease of the nipple. Usually the nipple becomes reddened. It may become thickened and hard or there may be a sore-like ulceration or erosion. When the nipple develops a sore like this your doctor should be consulted and a biopsy (removal of a piece of the nipple tissue) should be done to be studied under the microscope.
4. *Nipple discharge* Only five percent of nipple discharges (bloody) are associated with cancer. Most bloody nipple discharges are usually discovered by the patient. The color can be red, green, or black. The patient may notice it on the bed clothing or on her underclothing. Usually this is due to small growths within the ductal system of the breast that erode small blood vessels and cause the bloody discharge. You should see your doctor if this occurs. A clear yellow or white discharge from the breast is quite common and should not be confused with a bloody nipple discharge and is almost always benign.
5. *Redness to the skin or blotching* A rare form of cancer called inflammatory carcinoma can cause the skin of the breast to redden or become blotched as it would from infection or irritation. This is due to rapid growth of blood vessels within the tumor. If this condition persists it requires a biopsy for accurate diagnosis.
6. *Breast size* Compare the two breasts. If a breast suddenly increases in size and this can be seen or felt, it may mean that a cyst has formed and filled up with fluid or a solid growth may

have now become noticeable. If this is confirmed by "feel" then your doctor should be consulted. Many rapid increases in size of the breast are associated with cysts and often can be aspirated with a needle by your doctor and may not require surgery. If the breast has gotten smaller on one side, it may be due to puckering of the breast tissue in the deeper part of the breast by a growth and this should be investigated also.

7. *Armpit lump* The armpit is a common site for a lump to develop that may be involved with a tumor. This is where the cancer cells frequently drain to and this is where spread of a breast cancer can often occur. In fact, a woman can have a large lump under the armpit involved with a tumor and not be able to feel any lump in the breast tissue itself. In other words, one can have a very tiny cancer in the breast, not be able to feel it, and the first symptom that develops is a lump under the armpit. When this occurs, the doctor should be consulted and frequently a diagnostic work-up has to be done.

8. *Orange peel skin (peau-d'orange)* A peculiar orange peel appearance to the skin of the breast sometimes develops. This unusual enlargement of the pores and roughness of the skin texture on the breast, can be caused by a tumor that blocks channels carrying lymph fluid to and from the breast.

9. *Breast injury* Any injury to the breast can cause blood to accumulate under the skin (hematoma) or scarring and destruction of fatty tissue. This can result in a breast lump or swelling that may be confused with cancer. It can also cause difficulty in interpretation of an x-ray (mammogram). If the lump persists an aspiration biopsy should be done.

10. *Areola* Any noticeable variation, such as puckering or swelling, of the dark halo or areola that surrounds the nipple is a warning signal. It should be checked by a physician.

Breast Palpation In this technique, the patient lies down, places a small pillow or towel under the shoulder on the side of the breast to be examined and raises that arm above her head. What this does is to bring the breast tissue up on the chest wall so that the undersurface of the breast can be examined better (particularly in large busted individuals). It gives another approach to feeling the breast other than in the sitting or standing position. However, in some women, in the sitting position, when they lean forward, they can feel the contents of their breast better than in the supine or lying down position. The opposite palm of the hand, with the fingers closed, is used in palpating the breast, visualizing a clock with the upper portion of the breast at 12 o'clock and the lower portion of the breast at 6 o'clock. Next, examine the armpit by squeezing the fingers under the muscle and feeling for lumps. Then use the palm of the hand to firmly compress the breast tissue against the chest wall. At the lower curve of the breast, there is a ridge of firm tissue that is normal. Repeat the exam in a clockwise fashion but do not compress the tissue as firmly. This allows you to feel smaller subtle changes in the breast. The opposite breast is examined in a similar manner.

Upon completion of the palpable examination of the breast, the nipple and subareolar tissue (tissue under the nipple of the breast) is gently squeezed between the thumb and forefinger to see if there is any abnormal or bloody discharge from the nipple. If there is any, your doctor should be contacted. Here's what you should be looking for:

1. *Internal lumps* Most breast lumps are harmless—but new ones, particularly if hard or fixed, or old ones that grow, may indicate a tumor.
2. *Thickened tissue* Bands of thick, fibrous tissue that can be felt in the upper parts of heavy breasts and in the "shelving margin" underneath are a concern if they suddenly change in size.
3. *Breast contour* Any change in the contour or shape of the breast can be a warning sign as can puckering, swelling or dimpling.
4. *Nipple condition* Look for scaling, inversion, or discharge, either bloody or clear.
5. *Armpit lumps* The axilla (armpit) must also be palpated for growths, and this is often overlooked. In addition, the quarter of the breast closest to the armpit is the site of about half of all breast cancers.

Soaping the Breasts Many of my patients tell me they first found a lump while they were taking a bath or shower. This is not surprising since bumps and dips feel like mountains and craters under fingertips slick from soap or bath oil. Of course, what you are looking for are any of the symptoms already discussed.

WHEN ONE SHOULD NOT DO BREAST SELF-EXAMINATION

Some women are so nervous about their breasts that breast self-examination creates more problems than it's worth. Because of the publicity concerning cancer and the marked fear of cancer of the breast, some women cannot examine their breasts without becoming terrified and emotionally drained. These individuals would be better off by letting their doctors examine their breasts periodically. In some families in which cancer of the breast has occurred in a mother, aunt, grandmother, or even sister, it is impossible and impractical to teach these people breast self-examination. This type of patient is readily apparent in a doctor's office, since they constantly require reassurance.

WHAT IF YOU FIND A LUMP?

If you find something during your breast self-examination, don't panic. Rarely do swellings indicate the growth of new tissue, and even more rarely are they cancerous. If you have any doubts, most communities have specialists in the diagnosis and treatment of cancer. They can be found in the telephone directory under Oncology or Oncologists, or you can check with your local Medical Society for the names of cancer specialists nearest to you. The Cancer Information Service of the National Cancer Institute has a toll-free number you can call (800-638-6694) for current information on cancer specialists and hospitals, as do other organizations (listed in Appendix E).

If you have doubts concerning your diagnosis and treatment, you should seek a second opinion. The second opinion should be a physician or surgeon chosen by the patient and not someone recommended by the first doctor, who may be his buddy. The buddy system may prevent you from getting a good unbiased opinion. Sometimes, one has to go outside the local community to get a good unbiased second opinion.

In many cases, the diagnosis and treatment may be so difficult to determine, that a consensus opinion is necessary. This has led to Tumor Boards in large community hospitals, where many specialists combine to share their knowledge and opinions to help the breast cancer patient. A Tumor Board, however, is only as good as the people who serve on it.[13] The Board should have doctors serving on it who are true cancer specialists and should represent all the major disciplines that treat cancer patients. The members should include Medical Oncologists, Surgical

Figure 4
BREAST TUMOR SIZE AND DETECTION

Size of tumor seen on mammography
but cannot be felt

5 mm

Size of tumor first felt by
breast self-examination

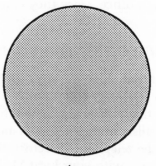

1 cm

Largest size of tumor
recommended for lumpectomy
(RX, controversial)

4 cm

If the tumor is this size
or larger, 50% will have
spread to other areas of
the body (metastases)

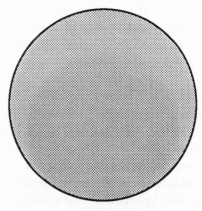

5 cm or larger

ACTUAL TUMOR SIZE

Oncologists, Radiation Therapists, Pathologists, and Immunologists.

Steady strides continue to be made against breast cancer and cancers of all types. Today, there are over a half-million women alive who have survived breast cancer, according to the American Cancer Society. Survival rates have increased even more dramatically in recent years as the result of breast self-examination and mammography. Moreover, it is becoming evident to everyone that breast cancer often is curable if diagnosed *and* treated early. See Figure 4.

This last dictum can't be overstressed. Among the patients in my survey, only half said they saw a doctor within one week of discovering a lump. Twenty percent waited three months or longer, and some took six months to a year before seeking any medical advice. Small wonder that in many of these patients, the cancer had spread outside the local area of the breast and in some, throughout the body.

The smaller the tumor size when detected, the more breast care options that are available to the patient.

3

The Medical Examination You Should Expect

Two of the major diseases that plague women are highly curable if they're caught early: cancer of the breast and cancer of the cervix. An annual checkup can detect the early stages of these cancers so they can be treated before they do serious harm. Yet more than half of all women fail to have a complete physical examination that includes a pap smear and examination of the pelvic organs and a good complete examination of the breasts that may or may not include a mammography.

The reasons they give for not having an examination are: they cannot be bothered, they are afraid of what may be found, and they cannot afford it.

If you're a woman who is among this majority it's important that you see a doctor once a year from now on—and particularly if you're over forty. If you are younger and have breast changes that are disturbing to you or to your doctor, you should have a baseline mammogram. This will provide a point of reference in case you develop a problem in the future. You should tell your radiologist that you want that mammogram saved for comparison in the future and if they are unwilling to save it, request that it be given to you since you paid for it and it's your breast and your life that you are trying to preserve.

A check-up for cancer requires a complete history and thorough physical examination. Your doctor should take a comprehensive history from you to determine if you fall into a high-risk group (Chapter 1), and whether or not a more extensive evaluation is needed together with a biopsy. Briefly, high-risk women are those who have: a family history of breast cancer, no children or children late in life, began menstruating early, northern European ancestry, and who are over thirty-five and overweight.

A good history by your physician will also include any previous surgery (for thyroid problems or other cancers), whether you have taken birth control pills or any kind of hormone preparation for menopausal symptoms, and which types of medications you may be taking (some can alter the structure or appearance of breast tissue). Biopsy results of previous surgery should also be added to your medical history as should any mammograms taken in the past.

The physical examination must include the skin, the breasts, the genital organs, and the organs of the chest, abdomen and reproductive system. A vaginal examination is essential, and no women should gamble with her health because of false modesty. Tell your doctor you desire a complete medical check-up. That should include a blood pressure check, electrocardiogram, height and weight, urine analysis, complete blood count, cholesterol, and other blood tests. Do not be alarmed if the doctor suggests other tests in addition to these. He may simply feel, as you do, that it is wise to take all precautions.

If you have rectal bleeding, he may suggest a proctosigmoidoscopy or colonoscopy and if he is unsure of what he feels on pelvic examination, an ultrasound of the pelvic organs may be ordered. Many new sophisticated tests are now available to the doctor to arrive at an accurate diagnosis.

Palpation and Biopsy Once a doctor has taken a complete history, he will examine your breasts using a method similar to that for breast self-examination. The patient disrobes and is first examined in the sitting position for any skin changes or bulges, nipple irregularities or discharge, and any difference in the size of the breasts. My experience has been that some breast conditions—bulges or dimples, in particular—can be more readily seen in a patient sitting or standing than when lying down.

Next the patient is told to lie down and the breasts are palpated for evidence of internal lumps or growths. The doctor should not be told where the patient has felt the lump so he will not be prejudiced in his own examination. The examination should also include palpation of the lymph glands in the adjacent armpit to see if they are enlarged or involved.

A stethoscope examination of the chest is then done to determine if the patient has any heart or lung problems. The abdomen is palpated and examined to see if the liver is enlarged, distended or nodular. The reason for this part of the examination is that estrogens, which have a lot to do with breast development, are detoxified in the liver and any damage to the liver such as in alcoholism may bring about changes in the breast tissue.

If the examination of the breasts reveals an obvious cyst (quite common), a needle aspiration can be done in the doctor's office under local anesthetic. The aspirated fluid can then be sent to a laboratory for analysis if it contains blood or cellular tissue. The patient is also advised to return in one month or sooner to be certain that the cyst does not refill or that there is no residual tumor present. In rare cases, a cancer can be next to a cyst or grow within the tissue wall.

Palpation, even by a doctor, can miss twenty percent of breast cancers—but used together with a biopsy that figure drops to less than one percent.

Needle Aspiration Needle aspiration is an inexpensive cost effective way of diagnosing breast tumors. In fact, it is the method of choice for many and can eliminate the anxiety that breast patients have waiting for a diagnosis. It can also be done in the doctor's office under local anesthetic to avoid the high cost of hospitalization.

Needle aspiration of a suspicious lump in the breast has been used as a diagnostic tool for sixty years. In 1925, Dr. Hayes E. Martin[14] of New York's Memorial Hospital routinely aspirated all palpable tumors. Thirty years later Dr. Otto Saphir,[15] used needle aspiration on breast lesions occurring in pregnancy and lactation to diagnose breast cancer. Today there is even less risk with the technique, and no evidence that tumor cells may be disseminated by the procedure.[16,17] New methods of preparing and preserving the tissue sample for cytological diagnosis have also been vastly improved.

The only problem is when needle aspiration is not done properly by other than a trained surgeon, a false result can be hazardous and lethal. The tumor can be missed and a false negative result can occur. The needle has to be directed in the proper place and enough tissue removed for diagnostic purposes. It may even be necessary to aspirate the suspected tumor in two or three different areas to obtain the correct sample.

The recently developed multihole needle for breast aspiration may solve this problem and appears to be less painful to the patient.[18]

Not all breast cancers can be diagnosed by needle aspiration, however, and cytological examination can sometimes give false positive results.[19] Scirrhous carcinomas, or stony tumors of the breast, are one example as are benign fibroadenomas or atypical histiocytes (scavenger cells present in connective tissue and lymph fluid). Inflammation and radiation effects on cell tissue can also make the diagnosis more difficult. When there is any doubt, needle aspiration should be followed by an open biopsy of the suspected tumor.

Open Biopsy In some large hospitals and cancer centers, needle aspiration is done more often than conventional open biopsy. However, my own feeling is that this practice is not without risks. First of all, there is an inherent danger in removing a breast (mastectomy) based solely upon a small sample of tissue taken through a needle. If you're having limited surgery or lumpectomy, there's no problem since the diagnosis is being confirmed and sufficient tissue is being obtained for further study.

In small hospitals, where aspiration techniques are limited and there are fewer cancer specialists, open biopsy should be done more often. In the past, a patient who went into a hospital for a breast biopsy often had her breast removed if the tissue sample proved malignant. This one-stage procedure is still the subject of great controversy and should not be done, particularly in young women with breast cancer. A two stage treatment method should be used.

No woman should have to wake up with her breast gone even if the biopsy shows she has a malignant tumor. It is far better to schedule an operation *after* the biopsy has been done and the physician can discuss with her the various treatment alternatives. This allows for full participation in the choice of treatment and means that she will be fully informed before giving her consent.

What About Mammography? Everyone agrees on the value of mammography (breast x-rays) in detecting tumors too small to be felt. What doctors, including myself, disagree on is when the benefits outweigh the risks of radiation exposure which in itself can cause breast cancer. Fortunately, newer machines deliver as little radiation to the breast as possible—less than one rad per mammogram in most cases and as little as 1/10 rad in some larger hospitals.

Few doubt the need or value of mammography for high-risk or older women, however, not all mammography (x-ray) equipment is monitored and calibrated regularly and the recommended dosages can be exceeded. Senator Jennings Randolph in Washington has been trying to get x-ray standards legislation passed for years. He is trying to get a bill passed that requires the government to set standards for certifying people other than doctors and dentists who administer x-rays. The West Virginia Democrat figured it would help prevent a dangerous situation. "There are many instances where people who give x-rays in hospitals and offices have no training." This can cause overexposure and serious health problems. Not all states in this country require x-ray machines in hospitals and medical offices be inspected. This should be done.

Radiation exposure is especially dangerous to young women and during pregnancy. Care must be taken so that the unborn child does not receive excessive radiation.

Sound clinical judgment is important in the evaluation of any breast cancer patient. No hard and fast answers can be given. I would suggest some guidelines for women to follow.

1. Monthly breast self-examination after age sixteen. (I have had patients detect breast lumps at this age.)
2. Breast examination by a doctor once a year after age forty.
3. Mammogram, if necessary, in the young female if lump is suspicious. (I have taken care of women with breast cancer at the age of 24 yrs.)
4. Screening mammogram at the age of 38 yrs.—for baseline study. Earlier age (35 yrs.) if woman falls into the high risk group.
5. Mammograms every year after age thirty eight, if woman falls into high risk group. Routine mammogram on low risk group every two-three years.
6. More frequent, and earlier, mammogram if there is a strong family history of breast cancer.

My own experience with mammography is that it should be done not only with women in the high-risk group, but those who have large breasts or who are overweight. To illustrate this point, consider the case of a woman, fifty-two, who was told by her doctor during a routine physical that she should have a mammogram. He said that her breasts were so large that he couldn't tell by palpation if she had a tumor.

The mammogram she had taken showed a calcium deposit beneath the nipple and deep within the breast. However, there was no recognizable lump. A biopsy was then arranged as a precaution and microscopic examination of the tissue sample did reveal a breast cancer. The patient was told the cancer was in an early stage and elected to have a lumpectomy and axillary dissection. During the operation the lymph nodes in the armpit were examined and showed no evidence of spread. The woman is alive today and her prognosis is excellent.

Why aren't more mammograms done? There is also the question of whether mass screening of the more than forty million women in this country for breast cancer is justified when the cost could exceed several billion dollars. Mammography should be selective, and the patient should be told there are alternative methods of detection that can provide similar results. Breast self-examination costs nothing and with practice any woman can find lumps as small as 3/4 inch or smaller.

Other Diagnostic Tests A special type of mammography called *xeroradiography*[20,21,22,23] can produce the same results as low dose x-ray mammography and the radiation exposure to the breast may be less. In this technique, the image of the breast is produced on a special coated paper, not on x-ray film. If you have to have frequent mammograms, you should insist that your radiologist inform you of the dosage you can expect during the study. You might also want to investigate some of the other diagnostic tests available:

THERMOGRAPHY[24,25,26] Infrared photography is used to measure the heat patterns coming from the breasts, detecting cancers because they are warmer than normal body tissues. It does not replace mammography or xeroradiography, but can be useful in screening women who are not at risk. False positive results could also lead to unnecessary biopsy or surgery.

ULTRASOUND High-frequency sound waves are projected into the breast to determine if a lump is solid (tumor) or a cyst. The technique is particularly helpful if the woman has large breasts or is apprehensive about needle aspiration. It is not as accurate as mammography, however. Ultrasound is also used to examine other areas of the body, including the kidneys, pelvis, pancreas, and uterus.

NUCLEAR MAGNETIC RESONANCE[27,28,29] The potential of this form of imaging has only recently been recognized. A large magnet with a hole big enough for a patient to fit through is surrounded by a radio-frequency transmitter. The images that are produced can pinpoint tiny breast cancers by detecting metal-bearing antibodies previously injected into the bloodstream. These concentrate at the tumor site where they are recorded by radiomagnetic signals. The technique shows promise but is still experimental and costly.

TRANSILLUMINATION This technique, also called diaphanometry, involves shining a light through the breast to outline its interior. Different types of tissues transmit and scatter the light in distinct ways, enabling doctors to more clearly perceive abnormalities. It is more commonly used to detect sinus problems and has only recently been investigated in the detection of breast cancer.

IMMUNOCYTOCHEMISTRY[30] Immunocytochemical techniques have now been developed to detect cancer cells that have spread from the breast to the lymph nodes in the armpit (the most common site). Monoclonal antibodies have been used and the technique is much more accurate. If the glands prove negative, no further treatment or surgery is necessary.

BLOOD TESTS It would be wonderful if we could take a sample of blood and, by studying it, determine whether or not a cancer was present in any part of the body. Unfortunately, medicine has not advanced this far. Blood tests are available, however, that can aid in the diagnosis of breast cancer by detecting certain proteins or other substances common in cancer patients. A specific blood test is helpful in determining whether breast cancer has spread or not. It is called the CEA antigen test.

SKIN TESTS A test similar to that used to detect tuberculosis is being evaluated. It is based on the fact that cells of breast tumors produce specific antigens to which the body should respond but doesn't. The tumor cells apparently escape detection by means of a "blocking factor" and continue to grow. This test has proved effective in detecting breast cancer in a number of cases.

RADIOISOTOPES Radioactive forms of iodine, gold, and other substances are now widely used in diagnosing cancer in certain organs, such as bone, liver, and thyroid gland. They tend to concentrate in specific areas, making it easier for doctors and radiologists to detect and diagnose tumors. Radiosotopes are particularly helpful in detecting whether a malignant tumor has spread to another organ.

RADIATION HAZARDS If radiation is used in the treatment of cancer, why worry about the effects of a single x-ray? First of all, no one is questioning the use of radiotherapy in the diagnosis and treatment of disease, including breast cancer. What specialists are worried about is the amount of exposure, how it is administered, and the damage to healthy tissues that may happen. Many Oncologists feel that excessive radiation can be just as damaging as radical mastectomy.

Dr. Nathan B. Friedman,[31] Clinical Professor of Pathology at the University of Southern California, has said that the permanent damage from radiation of normal breast tissue "ages it beyond its years and produces thin and atrophic (wasted away) skin and distended or spidery blood vessels that may require other treatment." Other studies [32,33,34,35] by several investigators have found evidence of breast cancer after x-ray treatment for postpartum mastitis (an inflammation of the breast caused by infection), pneumothorax therapy for tuberculosis, and in the survivors of Hiroshima who were young girls at the time and suffered no more than ten to fifty rads of radiation exposure. (A study done by the National Research Council[36] estimates that a dose of radiation above 120 rads doubles the chance of developing breast cancer and that the latency period can be as long as fifteen years.)

Another factor to take into consideration is the number of x-rays taken and the accuracy of the calibration equipment the radiologist or technician is using. A single exposure can be as much as 10 rads if several pictures are taken or more if the woman is nulliparous (no children) and the breast is hard to photograph, particularly if older x-ray equipment is used. The type of film used, the type of tube and filter, and the distance from the breast can also increase the total dosage to the patient. New equipment has reduced radiation exposure.

For these reasons, no one should have a routine x-ray. Routine, in this case, means without specific clinical reason and explanation. Without clinical evidence of its necessity, every x-ray you have adds to your total radiation exposure and presents hazards that can and should be avoided. The surgeon following young women in particular should be highly selective in doing mammography and suggest needle aspiration or biopsy as an alternative. Even in older women the risk of exposure has to be weighed against the possible long-term risks.

Any exposure to radiation is potentially harmful, since it can cause changes in normal cells as well as cancer cells. These changes occur in the genetic and protein-synthesizing components (DNA, RNA) of cells which are vital to our health. Frequent x-rays just add to the total amount of radiation the body receives and which remains in the cell tissue. Some diagnostic procedures in themselves have a high total dosage—barium enemas used in x-rays of the colon and intestines, and the newer computerized axial tomography (CAT) scans.

What Happens to My Tests? The importance of testing and analysis of breast cancer cannot be overemphasized. The American Cancer Society in *Cancer Statistics, 1985* reports an eighty percent cure rate when breast cancer is detected early. When it has spread, but not necessarily to distant sites, the figure drops to sixty percent. It also noted that only fifty-two percent of the cases of breast cancer were detected at this early, localized stage. In other words, half of the women who develop breast cancer are not getting optimal treatment because the cancer is not detected soon enough.

On the basis of the patient's history or self-examination, and the results of her physical examination by the doctor, it will be determined if further tests are necessary. Be sure you understand what they are and the directions for taking them as well as the results you can expect. Frequently the doctor will send you to a hospital, laboratory or radiologist's office for the tests.

To encourage hospitals to continually improve their anticancer efforts, the American College of Surgeons evaluates all hospital-based cancer programs. According to its *Cancer Program Manual,* the American Cancer Society is also attempting to encourage each hospital or institution to improve its cancer control efforts in the areas of prevention, early diagnosis, pretreatment evaluation, staging, optimal treatment, rehabilitation, and surveillance for recurrent and multiple primary cancer. For a current list of hospitals with approved cancer programs, you should contact the American Cancer Society (listed in Appendix E). There is no doubt that cancer programs in some hospitals are better than others. The strength of a cancer program is dependent upon the cancer specialists that work in that hospital and their training background.

Even though a doctor may be fairly certain from examination or x-rays that a tumor exists, it should be biopsied to see if it is benign or malignant. The tissue should be examined under a microscope by a pathologist. He may also use special stains to determine the structure and activity of the individual cells to see if they are cancerous and if so what type of cancer. Part of the tissue is also analyzed for estrogen and progesterone to determine if the cancer is hormone dependent. This information can be helpful in treatment if the tumor spreads or metastasizes. (See Appendix B)

If the tissue removed is of questionable nature, then it may be sent to another pathologist. The Armed Forces Institute of Pathology in Washington, D.C., maintains a diagnostic center to aid hospitals in obtaining a proper tissue diagnosis and these second opinions can be asked for by the patient. However, this is recommended only in the rare case in which a diagnosis is in question.

Summary/Questions Scientists do not know why certain women get breast cancer and others do not. We know that early detection reduces the chances of having that cancer spread, and makes it curable in most cases. If you find a lump during breast self-examination, see a doctor at once. Rarely are such lumps malignant. If you have any doubts about your doctor or your recommended treatment, remember, you are dealing with your own body, there are enough good physicians available for you to be choosy.

Not every woman will examine her breasts or see a doctor if she does find a lump. The fear of cancer bothers some more than others. There is no reason to run away from the idea, however. Face it squarely, and you will see it is actually far less terrible than most people imagine. Cancer can be treated successfully and can be curable. We do not know all about it, but we know a great deal. The answers to some of the questions that may bother you follow.

Q. *Will it hurt to have a needle aspiration?*
A. Not very much. The anxiety over having a needle stuck into the breast is too much for some women to bear, however, and a biopsy under general anesthesia may be worth considering.

Q. *Should you combine biopsy and surgery?*
A. No, the sample of tissue from the breast should always be thoroughly examined and this can take up to seventy-two hours depending upon the laboratory. This is much more definitive than the "frozen section" technique used in one-stage mastectomy.

Q. *Is there a best time for a mammogram?*
A. Not really, if you are over forty. Some radiologists prefer to do mammograms in relationship to the menstrual cycle. I find that the sooner it is done if they have a breast problem, the less anxiety they have.

Q. *What about older patients who need mammograms?*

A. They should have one every year, if they are in the higher risk group. You should consult your doctor about this, however. Most patients who have mammograms are apprehensive and it can help if the technician is female and takes time to fully explain the procedure.

Q. *Is there any evidence that radiation causes cancer?*

A. Yes, the Connecticut Tumor Registry, one of the largest in the world, reports that in a study of twins who were exposed prenatally to x-rays, the incidence of cancer was two to four times greater than those who were not.[37]

Q *How does needle localization differ from aspiration?*

A. The doctor uses a dye or hooked wire to pinpoint the growth in the breast before lumpectomy or other surgery. Most breast aspirations are done to eliminate cysts or as a preliminary diagnosis of cancer.

Q. *Can cysts develop into breast cancer?*

A. No, however, once a lump is diagnosed as a cyst, it is possible to become lax in breast self-examination. This should still be done once a month, every month.

Q. *Are some tumors harder to find than others?*

A. Yes, some breast tumors are not very cellular (atypical) and cytologists may miss them or give a false negative report. Scirrhous carcinoma of the breast is an example of such a tumor, and there are others.

4

Breast Lumps That Are Not Cancer

Most women will develop lumps in their breasts during their lifetime. The majority of the irregularities in the breast are related to hormone changes that occur with the menstrual cycle. Almost all lumps in the breast are benign and very few are changes that cause breast cancer. This does not mean that you should ignore these changes, rather you should be aware that they happen. Any lump that persists and does not go away should be investigated and you should see your doctor.

Thirty years ago, if a woman developed a lump in her breast that persisted, no matter what her age, she would have a biopsy to rule out cancer. There was no sophisticated imaging like mammography that could help the doctor accurately predict whether he might be dealing with a serious problem. The physician had to rely on what his fingers told him in examination of the patient. This led to extremes in anxiety for most women and fortunately, many times the doctor was wrong about the diagnosis—no cancer was found. Today, with mammography and aspiration biopsy techniques, we can accurately predict those patients that need a tissue biopsy.

Almost all breast problems in the younger age group are not malignant. Ninety-seven percent of my patients, under the age of thirty-eight years had no serious problems. Practically all of the women are

29

seen in the office, treated and discharged and not admitted to the hospital.

FIBROCYSTIC BREAST DISEASE

Fibrocystic breast disease is relatively common, occurring in fifty percent of women. It is the formation of benign cysts in the breast. Fibrocystic disease is exactly what it says. It is an area of fibrosis or thickening and an area of cystic change in the breast. The cysts can be multiple small cysts in which it is very difficult to obtain fluid or large multiple cysts which contain small or large amounts of fluid depending on the size of the cyst.

Although a cause or cure is unknown, some studies have shown that the distinctly lumpy or thickened areas within the breast are hormone-induced. They typically become more prominent before a menstrual period, and are most common in women aged thirty to fifty. The cysts that develop are rubbery, fluid fillled sacs that can become especially tender, even painful. The pain is often described as a dull ache unless the patient gets a sudden increase in size of a solitary cyst due to bleeding and then the pain can be quite severe.

If you have a history of cysts, you may have to have a needle aspiration to prove that the lumps are benign and contain fluid. This can be done in the office, under local anesthesia, sparing you the expense of a hospital stay, the risks of general anesthesia, and the anxiety of signing a consent form for a biopsy before you know what the lump is.

If you have a cyst that has been aspirated and contains fluid, be sure to see your doctor a month later to see if the cyst refills or residual tissue may be present. A biopsy sometimes has to be done since compression of a duct that contains a tumor can cause fluid to back up behind it. What this means is that even though a cyst is found, you should be religious about doing monthly breast self-examinations. Most patients with fibrocystic disease have several lumps in either one or both breasts and it is usually the patient who will first notice any change in the feel of their breasts.

Several years ago, it was thought that fibrocystic disease was a precursor to breast cancer. This is no longer the case several studies have shown.[38,39] In a review of all cases of proven fibrocystic disease in my own practice (500 cases) less than one percent went on to have a cancer of the breast.

FIBROADENOMAS

Fibroadenomas are a difficult problem to manage, more so than fibro-cystic disease. Fortunately fibroadenomas are not seen as often. They are firm solid lumps that develop in the young adult female and are fairly well circumscribed. They sometimes feel like an almond or pecan nut and can be multiple. Most of the time they are single lumps and small but sometimes they can be very large and almost replace the breast tissue.

Since fibroadenomas are solid tumors, if you try to aspirate them with a needle they don't contain fluid. If they occur in someone a little older they can be bothersome, since they have to be differentiated from cancer of the breast.

The surgeon has to be careful in removing a fibroadenoma, particularly if they are large and develop in a young woman. If you remove too much normal breast tissue, this can lead to underdevelopment of one breast and may eventually require plastic surgery.

INTRADUCTAL PAPILLOMAS

Papillomas are another type of growth within the breast, often occurring inside the duct near the nipple. They are too small to be felt, usually associated with a discharge, and common in women in their forties.

Intraductal papillomas usually present with a nipple discharge which is either pink, red, or greenish black in color. Compression of the nipple area in a clockwise fashion will usually indicate where the papilloma is and a discharge can be demonstrated. Ninety to ninety-five percent of intraductal papillomas are benign and malignancy is rare but does occur. The fact that malignancy does happen is a reason for excising all intraductal papillomas. Many of the papillomas are solitary and once they are excised, that's the end of the problem.

A case for illustration is presented: The patient is a forty year old white female seen in consultation with the chief complaint of bleeding from the left nipple of two weeks duration. A smear of the discharge was done by the family doctor and came back Class III. The positive findings were limited to the left breast. Compression of the nipple area in the ten o'clock axis produced a bloody discharge. Mammography studies were negative and at surgery, a small incision was made around the nipple and a dilated duct was located, a probe was passed and tissue removed. The duct was opened by the pathologist with the probe in place and a small papilloma was found that was benign. This patient is now sixty years of age and she has had no further difficulties.

MULTIPLE INTRADUCTAL PAPILLOMAS

Multiple intraductal papillomas are a much more dangerous problem than solitary papillomas and are more often associated with cancer. Papillomatosis is a precancerous lesion, as far as I'm concerned, and these patients have to be followed very closely. Mammography has to be done often and the patient should be seen more often in follow-up, since a breast cancer can develop in one of the intraductal papillomas.[40]

LIPOMAS

Lipomas are soft, benign tumors of the breast that consist of well differentiated fat cells. They can occur singly or in multiple nodules and usually never become malignant. In fact, a lipoma may suddenly stop growing when it is no more than an inoffensive little lump with a thin membrane around it.

Unfortunately, lipomas are solid lumps and sometimes are aspirated with a needle and since they don't contain fluid, may have to be operated on. Fortunately they are not cancer and the patient ends up happy. Do let your doctor check, if you find one. Only he can tell if a tumor is benign or malignant. Never decide for yourself "it's only a harmless growth."

DUCT ECTASIA

Duct ectasia is a term used to describe an inflammation of some larger ducts within the breast tissue. As a result of the inflammation, a nipple discharge can occur and fibrosis develops within the ducts that cause blockage of the glandular secretions that back up and form a lump under the nipple that may be palpable. Occasionally a serous, sticky or bloody discharge can occur and pain can also be associated with the lump. An advanced stage of duct ectasia or comedomastitis can develop which is inflammatory in reaction. The relationship of these lesions to cancer of the breast has not been determined.

OTHER REASONS NOT TO WORRY

There are several other variations of female anatomy that should not cause you any particular concern. Among them:

BREAST INJURY Such an injury will not cause cancer, either immediately or later in life. However, a very bad bruise can cause fat necrosis—breakdown of fat tissue—which may resemble a benign tumor. If such a lump, say from an automobile accident, remains after a reasonable length of time or seems to be growing in size, don't hesitate to see a doctor and have a biopsy.

UNUSUAL NIPPLES A dimple instead of a nipple is perfectly normal—if you've had one since puberty. Nipples that turn in later could be a sign of breast cancer. Consult your doctor. You needn't worry about an extra nipple, either. As many as seven percent of women have one, which may be mistaken for a mole. Simply cover it with makeup if you wish, or have the whole thing removed.

ASYMMETRICAL BREASTS One breast—usually the left—is often as much as ten percent larger than the other. If you're even more asymmetrical, or the change has only recently occurred, then you should see a doctor. It could be a cyst or papilloma that is responsible.

SUMMARY

Finding a lump in the breast is catastrophic to most women. The fear of cancer casts a shadow on lives which the disease itself will never touch. Those whom it does lay a hand on become so terror-stricken they are unable to fight back. Don't be one of them. Even though the enemy has not been wiped out, medicine is winning many battles.

If you find a lump, don't stick your head in the sand. Seek advice from a reputable doctor.

5

Pregnancy and Breast Problems

"Cancer"—the very word strikes fear in a woman's heart, especially if the disease threatens her reproductive system: breast, cervix, uterus, ovaries and vulva. It is one of the more difficult problems that face pregnant women and their doctors—but one that should not cause undue concern. Most lumps that occur during pregnancy are benign, and fewer than three women in one thousand will develop a breast cancer while pregnant.

The problem, if there is one, is that pregnant women or those who are breast feeding cannot do adequate breast self-examination. It is also difficult for the obstetrician to detect any changes in the breast—particularly in the second and third trimesters of a pregnancy. If the woman is obese to start with or has large breasts, the problem is compounded. Because of this, the physician has to be aggressive in the diagnosis of breast cancer during pregnancy.

DETECTION AND TREATMENT

The most important consideration for patient and obstetrician is to try to detect the cancer *early*. Simply feeling the engorged breast and swollen belly is no longer adequate. When a woman is pregnant she should do breast self-examination, even though it may be more difficult. If any changes are noted in the breast and the doctor confirms it, the new imaging diagnostic techniques, such as mammography, should be used. Since most imaging methods use radiation, it is possible to protect the unborn baby by putting a lead shield over the mother's abdomen, and this is done routinely in most hospitals.

The main objective in the treatment of pregnant women with breast cancer is to cure the patient and deliver a healthy baby. This can only be done if the cancer is localized and detected before it spreads to the axillary (armpit) nodes or other organs. However, because of unfounded fears on the part of patient and doctor alike, this is not always the case. Three-fourths of the pregnant patients with breast cancer in one study had metastases (spread) to the axillary nodes requiring surgery.[41]

Another point to consider when taking tests is that pregnancy in itself suppresses the body's immune system and causes a decrease in the cancer fighting lymphocytes present in the blood.[42] This change is due in part to the influence of hormones, which greatly increase during the second and third trimester. My initial approach when a lump is found during pregnancy is to aspirate the lump with a needle to see if it contains fluid (benign cyst) and to take a small piece of tissue for analysis. This can be done under local anesthetic with little or no discomfort to the patient.

If the woman is apprehensive about the needle, she can be given intravenous Valium or some other medication so that she will relax during the procedure.

The following example illustrates the difficulty in diagnosing breast cancer when the features of pregnancy mask or cause problems for the physician:

A thirty-year-old woman having her first pregnancy was told she was pregnant when in her third month. A physical examination indicated she was healthy and she was advised by the obstetrician concerning medications and nutrition. At six months a member of the group practice examined her and detected a small lump in her right breast. She was then told to see a general surgeon who also examined her and arranged for monthly visits until she went to full term, which she did.

By then her breasts had enlarged and further examination to see if the lump had increased in size were futile. She delivered a normal, healthy baby and she asked if she could breast feed the child. She was told to do so by both the obstetrician and surgeon who examined her. After three months of breast feeding the lump in her right breast became quite obvious, and a biopsy was suggested. It revealed an infiltrating ductal breast cancer that had spread to five lymph nodes in the armpit and which required a modified mastectomy and axillary dissection.

RISKS TO THE CHILD

The case history cited underscores several points that should be considered when a woman develops breast cancer during pregnancy. The most important of these is that diagnostic tests for breast cancer early in pregnancy present little or no risk to the unborn child. Second, if the cancer is detected during the second or third trimester, the prognosis is poorer than it would be during the first trimester.[43]

Pregnant women with breast cancer have been successfully treated with drugs during their pregnancy and delivered healthy babies with no evidence of toxic effects.[44,45] Others have had a simple biopsy or lumpectomy to remove a breast tumor and went on to give birth with no injury to mother or child. One should be careful of the drugs that are used, however, since some of them can cause birth defects.

As to whether the pregnancy should be terminated if a woman develops breast cancer, there are no hard and fast answers. The question of abortion aside, it would depend upon the stage of the cancer and whether or not the woman already had one or more healthy children. In the latter case, my own advice would be to terminate the pregnancy in the first trimester and treat the cancer. If this is not possible, the mother and child could be monitored (mammography and ultrasound) and the baby delivered early or by caesarean section. This would permit aggressive chemotherapy, if needed, for the mother at an earlier date.

The time to detect breast cancer is early, when it is still small and localized. If physicians don't conduct the necessary tests and patients don't know enough to request them, pregnant women will continue to risk their health and possible loss of their breasts.

SHOULD YOU BREAST FEED?

Contrary to what's been believed for many years, breast feeding is not reliable as a natural means of preventing breast cancer. Studies indicate, in fact, that a percent of nursing mothers develop breast cancer and that the percentage rises significantly for women in the higher risk groups.[46]

There's also the risk to the mother of increased hormones in the breast milk, which have been shown to promote the growth of breast tumors in several studies. It is known, for example, that plasma pro-lactin levels increase during lactation as do the levels of estrogen and progesterone.

Prophylactic removal of the ovaries is not necessary after childbirth in women with breast cancer, however, since it has not proved to be an effective means of cure or increasing survival.[47,48] The treatment in lactating women should be the same as that for women who aren't pregnant or who have had children in the past.

WHAT ABOUT DES?

Before the Food and Drug Administration took action on diethylstil-besterol (DES) about four million women used the drug during preg-nancy in order to prevent miscarriage. A recent study in the *New England Journal of Medicine* shows a forty-seven percent greater risk of breast cancer for these women.[49]

The daughters of these DES users, many of them now in their child-bearing years, are also believed to have twice the risk of developing dysplasia and carcinoma in situ (both precancerous conditions) and they should consult with their physician so that they may be watched at more frequent intervals. These women are at greater risk to develop vulvar cancer as well as cancer of the cervix.

A Pap test can be taken from these anatomical areas. The Pap test is a routine method of collecting cells from the cervix, having them ana-lyzed, and then determining whether or not abnormal cell changes are taking place. It has saved the lives of millions of women. The cure rate for cervical cancer is approaching one hundred percent in the forty years since the Pap test was introduced.

SUMMARY/QUESTIONS

Only a small number of doctors meet all the guidelines in testing for breast cancer suggesting either unfamiliarity with them, or an exag-gerated concern for the patient's reluctance to undergo the tests. Either reason fails to justify the breach. No woman, particularly one who is pregnant, should have to fear for her life or that of her child. An informed patient can help her doctor by pointing out that she is past a given age or at higher risk. Any doctor who brushes the suggestion aside is then inviting the patient to find another doctor.

Q. *Are most lumps that develop during pregnancy malignant?*

A. No, the majority are benign. A woman can develop any type of breast problem when she is pregnant as when she is not pregnant.

Q. *Are there tests other than mammography for detecting breast cancer?*

A. Yes, but not all are as accurate. Among them are thermography, ultrasound, nuclear magnetic resonance and transillumination (discussed in Chapter 3).

Q. *How accurate is needle aspiration of the breast?*

A. It depends, if it is done by a skilled surgeon familiar with the technique and an adequate sample is taken; and the laboratory has good cytopathologists, the tissue analysis can be ninety percent accurate.

Q. *Can anyone take my mammogram?*

A. Yes, but they shouldn't. The pictures of your breast are only as good as the person reading them and that should be a trained radiologist. There is also the added risk of overexposure by an untrained specialist or nurse unfamiliar with the x-ray equipment.

Q. *Should a woman who has had a mastectomy get pregnant?*

A. There's no reason not to, if she is young and willing to wait a while to be certain there is no recurrence. No waiting period is necessary for a noninvasive cancer (lobular carcinoma, for example).

Q. *Is it more difficult to detect a breast lump when a woman is pregnant?*

A. It depends when the breast lump or tumor develops. If a woman develops a tumor in the first trimester of her pregnancy, it usually is not difficult to determine clinically that there is something wrong within the breast tissue. A malignant tumor is usually firmer, probably not tender and may be attached to underlying muscle or skin. However, if a tumor develops later in the pregnancy, when the breasts are larger, it is much more difficult to clinically decide if a problem exists.

Q. *If a pregnant woman develops a breast cancer in the sixth month (later half) of her pregnancy, is it more dangerous to her than in the first trimester (first three months)?*

A. If a woman develops a breast cancer during the second half of her pregnancy, she has a poorer prognosis than one who develops a cancer during the first half of her pregnancy.[43] Most patients who develop breast cancer during the second half of their pregnancy show evidence of spread of their cancer to lymph nodes and this suggests that they are in an advanced stage of their disease. This automatically means that they are at greater risk.

Q. *What if a breast lump is detected immediately after birth of a child and the mother is breast feeding? If it's cancerous is it more dangerous? In other words, if the mother is lactating and she develops a breast cancer is the survival rate poorer?*

A. There are some who feel that lactation reduces the risk of breast cancer despite findings to the contrary in some studies.[46] I have seen lactating women with breast lumps and if the size of the breast is large it can be extremely difficult to detect a cancer in this type of breast and this can lead to delay. If there is prolonged delay in diagnosis and treatment, of course the survival rate will be poor.

Q. *What is the best treatment for cancer of the breast in a pregnant patient?*

A. When a malignant tumor develops in the breast of a pregnant patient, the diagnosis and treatment methods should be the same as the woman who gets cancer of the breast when she is not pregnant. If radiation diagnostic techniques are used, the fetus should be protected from radiation exposure.

Q. *What are the five and ten year survival rates for a woman who becomes pregnant following a mastectomy?*

A. The same as for women who do not become pregnant. Again, each case has different factors that must be weighed, including age, health and type of surgery.

6

Are Hormones Really to Blame?

Estrogens are female hormones produced by the ovaries. They are largely responsible for the changes that take place at puberty in young girls. By their direct action they cause the development of the breasts through the formation of breast ductal growth. They also cause the growth and development of the vagina, uterus, and fallopian tubes. During a normal menstrual cycle, estrogens stimulate the breasts to enlarge and a fullness of the breasts develops.

Estrogens are also made in the placenta and adrenal glands and also can be made in the liver and skeletal muscle from other steroid hormone precursors.

In the natural course of a woman's life, as menopause approaches, all women experience a decrease in estrogen production. As the amount of estrogens decrease in the blood some women develop symptoms related to the menopause, however, many do not. The majority of women go through the menopause without any problems. Hot flashes and atrophic vaginitis associated with dryness and painful intercourse can develop and interfere with the normal lifestyle of the female.

When this happens some doctors will routinely put them on replacement therapy (estrogens). Estrogen, touted as the "feminine forever" drug, was one of the most frequently prescribed drugs of the early seventies. Millions of menopausal women received estrogen to restore

40

their hormonal balance and relieve the distress that sometimes accompanies the change of life.

The estrogen replacement therapy worked, but then a series of studies[52,53] found that women taking the drug for prolonged periods—more than two years—had four to eight times greater chance of developing cancer than did women who never received the hormone. For many menopausal women it was a fearful discovery: Estrogen's risks suddenly appeared greater than any benefits. When this adverse alarming fact became known to the public, the drug manufacturers added progestin to help neutralize the estrogen effect and hopefully decrease the risk for cancer.

Many news media articles have stated that the risk of cancer has been lessened, but insuffucient time has elapsed to determine who may be right. Indiscriminate hormone replacement with high dose estrogen has been shown to promote tissue growth in human breast tissue[54] and this has been also established in research on experimental animals.[55] Other studies have linked high estrogen levels in women in high risk groups to develop cancer of the uterus.[56,57,58,59]

ESTROGENS AND THE MENOPAUSE

The use of estrogens at the menopause and the effect of estrogens on the breast tissue to produce a breast cancer has been a matter of controversy in medical circles for years. The increased risk has been noted by the National Institutes of Health and no one knows what the long term effects might be. Apparently the longer you take estrogen, the greater the risk. Which is why, women and physicians should take a much closer look at what, for years, has been an accepted practice.

Even today, more than seven million women past menopause are taking estrogen supplements. Why? Aside from relieving some menopausal symptoms, they erroneously believe that estrogen will keep them looking young, prevent their breasts from sagging and increase their life expectancy. There is simply no evidence that estrogen will do any of these things. There is, however, firm evidence that prolonged use of estrogen *will* increase the risk of breast cancer.

Doctors who routinely prescribe estrogen supplements are not allowing the body's natural physiological mechanisms to adapt to the change going on. Menopause is not a single event but a process that takes place over about fifteen years—from about the age of forty-five to sixty.

The first missed period is definitely not a signal of menopause. So, forget whatever myths you may have heard about negative effects of "the change" and seek a second opinion before starting estrogen therapy. More likely than not, the only change you will notice is one for the better.

Only ten to fifteen percent of menopausal women really need treatment. Many can benefit from alternative therapies. For example, to relieve vaginal dryness you can use a water-soluble lubricant during intercourse. Brittle bones (osteoporosis) will respond to a diet high in calcium and protein and vigorous exercise can help maintain bone strength.

With all that's written about what to do about the problems of menopause, we sometimes tend to forget that the vast majority of women pass through this period without a major problem and require no treatment and no medication. For those who don't, there are many more safe alternatives to estrogen. So don't hesitate to discuss them with your gynecologist or family doctor. Even when the doctor prescribes estrogens (typically after induced menopause or hysterectomy), you should be concerned about the dosage and length of treatment.

QUESTIONS

Q. *What should a woman do if she develops hot flashes at the menopause and has difficulty tolerating them?*

A. She should see her physician first. There are many methods that aid in controlling hot flashes other than estrogens. Tranquilizers can be used. Support by the physician at this time is helpful also. If it is necessary to use estrogens, minimal doses only should be used and close follow-up by the physician should be done to be sure that adverse side effects do not occur.

Q. *How long should a woman continue to take estrogens?*

A. Each case has to be individualized. There has to be a cut-off time, however. I recently saw a patient with breast cancer eighty-one years of age who was still taking estrogens and she had not seen her gynecologist for fifteen years.

Q. *Are there some women who should not be given estrogen supplements?*

A. Yes there are. Estrogen supplements should not be used in those females that have severe liver disease (alcoholics and cirrhotics, for instance), also patients with blood clotting disorders or severe heart disease. Estrogen is inactivated mainly in the liver and if the liver is damaged, retention of excessive estrogens occurs. A small amount of estrogen is excreted in the bile and is reabsorbed from the intestines. The liver is involved in blood clotting mechanisms and the indiscriminate use of estrogens in these patients can be hazardous to their health.

Q. *Some women seem to breeze through the menopause with minimal symptoms and others seem to have difficulty with severe hot flashes. Why is that?*

A. Vasomotor flushes or sweats are poorly understood symptoms and not all women get them. They eventually will subside without treatment.

Q. *What should you do if you feel that you absolutely need estrogen therapy?*

A. To reduce the risks of getting cancer, estrogen therapy, if given at all, should be given in conjunction with progestins. In those women who are in the high risk group for breast cancer, hormone therapy should not be given at all to the postmenopausal women, unless absolutely necessary and should not be given to women who have cancer of the reproductive organs.

Q. *What if a woman has to have a hysterectomy and oophorectomy early in life and needs replacement therapy?*

A. Women who have hysterectomies early in life and are in the high risk group for breast cancer, should be very carefully watched if they are on replacement estrogen therapy and the level of estrogens should be minimal and should be given with progestins.

Q. *If a woman has a hysterectomy and oophorectomy (ovary removal), will she be protected from getting breast cancer?*

A. Seventeen percent of my breast cancer patients had hysterectomies and oophorectomies and then took replacement therapy. It is obvious that it did not protect these women from getting breast cancer.

Q. *How does a doctor advise a patient as to whether she should take estrogens, particularly since the risk factors may outweigh the benefits?*

A. The decision has to be made by the patient and the doctor. It definitely has to be individualized. The woman must be absolutely sure that she is getting accurate information. It is a personal decision in which the doctor must express his opinion as to the state of the art of the treatment at the time the decision is made. To make this choice intelligently, the woman must be given all the information available about the positive and negative effects of the use of estrogens. It should also be remembered that some patients require estrogens for necessary medical reasons.

THE BIRTH CONTROL PILL

The recent twenty-fifth anniversary of the birth control pill has been embraced by its manufacturers as an occasion to mount a publicity campaign to tell women the Pill is safer than ever. How much of this hoopla is hype? The sensitive response should be healthy skepticism. For while the Pill remains unsurpassed for convenience and effectiveness, the question of its safety persists.

In fact, the question most asked about the birth control pill is the same one posed years ago: "Does the Pill Cause Cancer?" The answer to that is not a clear yes or no. A number of studies begin to give us some definitive answers. One of these, done in Los Angeles by British Dr. Malcolm C. Pike,[60] did show an increased rate of breast cancer in young women taking birth control pills. However, since most women studied until now have been in their fifties (when the Pill contained large amounts of estrogen), the cause-and-effect relationship to breast cancer is not clearcut. A controversy is still present as to whether the birth control pill increases or decreases the risk of getting breast cancer. Research in this area is extremely difficult to do because of so many variables that have been introduced.

During the past twenty years there has been a change in the chemical make-up and potency of the Pill. Both the estrogen and progestogen steroids present in the Pill have decreased. In 1964, ninety-two percent of the Pills marketed contained more than 50 meg. of estrogen. By 1983 only nine percent of the Pills prescribed had more than 50 meg. of estrogen and fifty-two percent had less than 50 meg. of progestogen.[60,61]

A word about birth control. The way the Pill works is by altering the body's hormonal balance so that the ovaries do not produce the eggs necessary for fertilization. There is also a thickening of the mucous lining of the uterus which prevents the sperm from fertilizing any egg that is produced. The latter is caused by progestin (a form of progesterone) present in both the combined and so-called "mini" pills.

Taking the Pill also increases the rate of cell division in the lobules of the breast, which is what happens in the growth of a cancerous tumor.[62] Studies have also shown that progesterone can cause breast hyperplasias (considered as precancers) and lobular carcinomas when taken in large doses or for extended periods of time.[63] This is particularly true for "first-generation" birth control pills that women began taking in the sixties, and which contained more estrogen.

There is also evidence that women who have never had children are at greater risk of developing breast cancer. So, the longer a woman waits to have her first baby, the less opportunity there is for the natural protective effect of pregnancy and lactation.[64] What this means is that young women who take the Pill and have never been pregnant lack an adequate response to the progesterone (the antagonist to estrogen in the Pill). This female will, in effect, be exposing her breasts to unopposed estrogen and will be placing her breasts at increased risk to getting breast cancer.[65] The following case history demonstrates this effect on the body's normal defense mechanisms:

A young woman, twenty-four, was examined and a lump found in her right breast which a mammogram confirmed as cancerous. She had been taking the Pill for five years beginning at seventeen, and stopped in order to get pregnant. The medications she then received to regain her normal menstrual cycle contained a high dose of estrogen and progestin. She did not regain a normal menstrual cycle and the lump persisted and biopsy was done.

It revealed an invasive ductal cancer of the breast and nipple and she was admitted to the hospital for further diagnostic testing. The liver scan showed extensive spread of the cancer and treatment was begun. However, because of the advanced stage of her breast cancer, the woman died four months after her initial biopsy.

COMPLICATIONS OF THE BIRTH CONTROL PILL

Many adverse side effects developed from the use of the early Pill; strokes, heart attacks, severe migraine headaches, phlebitis, diabetes, and cancer. Most of these adverse side effects were related to either the estrogen or progestin content in the pill and specific research documented these problems.

The vascular changes occurred most frequently and are probably related to the progestin dose in the Pill. If progestogens are added to the Pill, there seems to be an added coronary risk. Estrogens seem to decrease this risk.

BIOPSY AND BENIGN BREAST DISEASE

If the apparent link between the Pill and breast cancer is confirmed, it will be particularly bad news for women with benign breast disease or fibrocystic disease—a condition that may cause discomfort but in no way threatens a woman's life or overall health. The Pill has been shown to prevent benign breast disease and to shrink or eliminate breast cysts around the time of ovulation by suppressing the normal hormonal cycle that causes them to appear.[66,67] This condition is most common in younger women but should not indicate a biopsy is routinely necessary—even in those women who are not on the Pill.

In fact, the incidence of biopsies for benign breast disease has greatly decreased in recent years with the advent of imaging techniques (mammography) and more frequent breast self-examination. Those that are done are also more meaningful and have helped to cut down the rate of needless surgery. There's really no reason for a woman with fibrocystic breast disease (discussed in Chapter 4) to be unduly concerned that she will get breast cancer if the condition persists.

SUMMARY/QUESTIONS

The Pill *is* safer than it was, because the estrogen dosage has been substantially reduced. It may even have some benefits to some users. There is little doubt about the link between estrogen and breast cancer especially in women who take the Pill for long periods of time. Until more studies are done, it's up to each woman to reach her own decision based on the evidence.

Q. *What if you want to take the Pill?*
A. Don't if you smoke or are over thirty-five. In any case, watch carefully for any danger signals: blood clots, pain in the abdomen, numbness in the arm, or growths in the breast.

Q. *Are there any benefits to taking the Pill?*
A. Yes, aside from preventing benign breast disease, the Pill has been shown to lower the incidence of pelvic inflammatory disease (PID), which is a common cause of infertility. It has also reduced the rate of iron-deficiency anemia caused by long menstrual periods and excessive blood loss.

Q. *Can taking the pill affect any medical tests?*

A. Yes, thyroid function tests can be affected, as can blood glucose and plasma insulin tests.

Q. *Should women taking the Pill have other tests?*

A. Definite monthly breast self-examination is a must, as is an annual check-up. Routine Pap smears should also be done and the abdomen palpated (for evidence of liver enlargement).

Q. *Did any of your breast cancer patients take the Pill?*

A. Yes, fifteen to seventeen percent of my patients who developed breast cancer were on the birth control pill and still got breast cancer. Many of these women took the pill when it contained high doses of estrogen. This suggests that the birth control pill does not protect you from getting breast cancer.

Q. *Do you feel that the birth control pill causes cancer?*

A. I don't think anybody can answer that question. I have tried to point out some of the beneficial and harmful effects of the Pill. There is no doubt that the Pill has been improved. One of the biggest problems is to try and define those women who would be at increased risk if they take the Pill. I believe this problem can be solved in the future. There is no doubt that some women are hurt by the Pill. It may take many years and a few generations to determine the long term effects of the Pill; that is, whether it is good or harmful.

7

Informed Consent

Just what is informed consent for the breast cancer patient prior to treatment? How does the doctor explain the various methods of treatment and the results of that treatment since there now are so many options and so many controversies concerning the results of each treatment?

Who should define what the best treatment is? Some of the best minds in research and some of the best clinical cancer specialists cannot agree on how the breast cancer patient should be treated. Because of the magnitude of the breast cancer problem (120,000 new breast cancer cases diagnosed each year) the news media has capitalized on the attention of the problem and in some cases has prejudiced the patient concerning treatment methods; patients come into the doctor's office, all expecting to have their breasts saved if they have breast cancer.

Some of these patients do not qualify for breast conservation surgery. As has been stated previously in this book, approximately half of the breast cancer patients when first diagnosed have evidence of spread of their cancer (regional lymph node metastases) or systemic metastases[1] and should not have minimal surgery. Other methods are used to try to save their lives and give them a quality of survival.

Informed consent means exactly what it says. It means that the patient wishes to be fully informed or instructed comprehensively about her options in treatment in order to select the method that she wants to be used on her. After being fully informed, if that is possible, she then consents to the treatment.

She may also decide to refuse the treatment or seek a second opinion from a recognized trained cancer specialist. This means that if the patient is mentally alert, she is allowed to consult and to agree to the treatment to be used on her body or to refuse. In other words, she is the captain of her own destiny.

In some cases it is almost impossible to clearly explain anticipated treatment methods and the numerous options particularly if something more than a segmental resection (lumpectomy) is to be done on the patient. This is due to the emotional stress and anxiety associated with the discovering of the breast lump.

Only a small percentage (10–15%) of women qualify for limited surgery to preserve the breast. In many cases the recommended treatment is a modified mastectomy and axillary dissection because of the size of the tumor and the stage of the disease or the tissue diagnosis.

Some states have passed laws requiring informed consent for the breast patient (California, Massachusetts, Hawaii, and Wisconsin). Other states are now considering passage of informed consent laws. These laws have introduced additional medico-legal problems for the doctor in the treatment of the breast cancer patient and has increased the cost of care. Some states require the physician to discuss all the options of treatment and possible complications and risks associated with the method chosen (New York, Vermont). This means that the risks explained to the patient must conform to the practice and treatment methods of the medical profession in that community.

This assumes that the treatment methods in that community are good for the patient and that there is some conformity to the treatment methods that are practiced nationally at the major cancer research centers.

Not all major cancer research centers or hospitals treat breast cancer the same way, however. Breast cancer is currently treated by several different methods. Each case of breast cancer has to be individualized. Every woman should discuss, with their cancer specialist, all the options available and the reasons for the specific procedure being done on them. There is no one approach suited to the needs of all patients with breast cancer. In this book I have tried to discuss the various breast care options that are available and some of the possible risks associated with those treatment options.

The treatment methods used are the state of the art at that time and may be completely different twenty years later. A prime example is the treatment of breast cancer. Radical mastectomy has been the treatment of choice for 60–70 years. Today, approximately four percent have this method of treatment.

One of the biggest breakthroughs that has affected the treatment methods during the past twenty years has been the ability to detect minimal cancers by the use of imaging devices (mammography, xeromammography, and ultrasound) which means that because the cancer is very small we can now offer the patient many different options in treatment.

This means that there are many different modalities that can be recommended for primary curable breast cancer. This includes segmental resection (lumpectomy) with lymph node dissection, and/or radiation therapy, modified or total mastectomy and axillary dissection or radical mastectomy or extended radical mastectomy with or without radiation, etc.

In the future, there will be many more sophisticated new methods of treatment advocated. The passage of time usually determines whether a method is good or bad.

In many institutions, long legal forms are used prior to anticipated treatment of the breast cancer patient. I have seen some of these forms and the legal verbiage used can only lead to more confusion on the part of the patient.

Prominent lawyers have told me that the informed consent form means nothing. Once you get into the courtroom all the patient has to state is that she didn't understand.

Many patients seek second or third opinions when they have a serious breast problem. Often these second and third opinions are in conflict with each other, which leads to further confusion for the patient.

An average level of intelligence is necessary on the part of the patient in order for the patient to select a treatment method that they can live with and be satisfied with. Not all patients have this level of intelligence. There is a futility that occurs and there is a definite difficulty in trying to explain everything to the patient.

It is impossible to inform the patients completely about what will happen to them following the selected treatment. To emphasize this point, I would like to give two examples about the unpredictability of breast cancer.

The first is a woman of fifty-nine years of age who had a breast cancer treated with mastectomy. Ten years after her mastectomy she developed a severe toothache and saw an oral surgeon who, while doing a root canal, noted some peculiar tissue in the tooth socket. She had no other symptoms. The tissue from the tooth socket was sent to the laboratory and a diagnosis of metastatic breast cancer was made. Except for this area of involvement, there was no evidence of bone, liver, or soft tissue spread. Four months later evidence of diffuse systemic spread developed.

The second case was a thirty-five-year-old white female, who also had a mastectomy for breast cancer, and two years later noted blurring and a blind spot in her vision. An ophthalmologist was able to diagnose a spread of the breast cancer to the retina and choroid of the eye. A few months later evidence of diffuse systemic spread developed in this case also.

These two cases demonstrate how it is impossible to determine how breast cancer will present itself at a later date. No consent form could predict this outcome.

Does the surgeon or breast cancer specialist have to guarantee that the breast cancer patient will get a good result from their treatment and be cured or be restored to good health? The answer is no.

Not all patients are healthy vigorous individuals and you cannot always predict the outcome. Not all patients eat a good healthy diet, have regular exercise, and see their physician regularly for their health problems. Delay in diagnosis and treatment is not uncommon with breast cancer. The patient is partially to blame for that, for many women do not do breast self-examination on a regular basis and do not get a mammogram when it is recommended.

Should the patient be told that there may be delayed risks to their treatment? If a lumpectomy is done followed by radiation therapy; there may be a higher incidence of local recurrence after ten or fifteen years. The damage to the chest wall and the breast by radiation could possibly induce a cancer that may occur fifteen to twenty-five years after treatment. Is delayed recurrence after radiation treatment most important or total survival of the patient and preservation of the breast?

Many times the patient participates in the discussion of her options and chooses to save her breast even though the risk factors may be higher. Not all of these patients are able to preserve their breasts when a recurrent cancer develops and the patient's decision may be the wrong one.

The question can be asked as to whether the patient should be told about delayed failure of the many surgical methods. Not all the risks, complications, or recurrences can be anticipated. Not all surgery is the same and not all surgeons have the same amount of expertise.

INFORMED CONSENT CONCERNING SURGICAL COMPLICATIONS

Whenever a patient has an operation and a general anesthetic is used, there is always a small risk associated with doing the operation. Since the breast is more or less a surface organ there is not as much risk in doing the operation on the breast as there might be with a complicated resection of organs, such as kidney, colon, or stomach. Complications still occur, however, and not all patients are in good health prior to their operation.

SURGICAL COMPLICATIONS

Breast surgery, no matter what type is done, is not without its complications and this has to be discussed with the patient. Since fewer radical procedures are now being done and simpler surgical procedures have taken their place, complications have decreased dramatically.

The younger patients have fewer complications than the older patients and this should be expected. Wound healing is poorer in the older age group and sometimes skin grafts are needed. Fluid collection under the skin flaps can occur, although with the new suction devices to withdraw this fluid, they are less frequent. Occasionally an infection will develop but antibiotic therapy usually handles the problems.

Radical mastectomy is not done often today and therefore, lymphedema of the arm on the side of removal of the breast is infrequently seen. We no longer see limitation of motion of the shoulder and the cosmetic defect created by radical mastectomy, when the chest wall muscles are removed.

Modified mastectomy (removal of the breast tissue without the muscles) and axillary dissection (glands in the axilla-armpit) is done most often at the present time, although segmental resection and axillary dissection followed by radiation is on the increase.

When these conservation breast procedures are done a question frequently asked by the patient is; Did I do the right thing and did the limited surgery and radiation destroy the cancer? That issue is addressed in the next two chapters on treatment.

INFORMED CONSENT AND RADIATION THERAPY

Radiation therapy has usually been considered an adjunctive method of treatment for breast cancer and not as a primary method of treatment.

This concept has changed with a greater percentage of breast cancers being detected when they are small minimal cancers and cannot be felt in the breast.

Radiation therapy is now being used as a primary treatment of breast cancer following segmentectomy (lumpectomy) and axillary dissection to attempt to sterilize the local resected area from residual cancer cells. A higher dose radiation is now being used and a more sophisticated technique is being done.

It is too early to determine the results of this method of treatment but there are many advocates for the use of this method since it does preserve the breast. Complications can develop from the use of this treatment method however.

Since higher dose radiation is being used, the patient has to be fully informed of the possible complications or delayed consequences of their treatment.

Rib fractures and lymphedema of the arm can occur and radiation pneumonitis and sometimes neurological deficits can develop, such as motor weakness to the hand or arm. Radiation damage to the brachial plexus can be quite debilitating. Fortunately, it does not occur often.

In some sections of the country, segmentectomy (lumpectomy) and axillary dissection is being done without radiation therapy. These patients also have to be informed of the possible increased risk of local recurrence.

INFORMED CONSENT AND CHEMOTHERAPY

Not all patients are fortunate enough to first present to their doctor with localized disease of the breast. In the report on the 1982 National Survey of Carcinoma of the Breast,[1] one half of the patients (52%) were diagnosed in the localized stage of the disease, while 38% were diagnosed in the regional stage with axillary node involvement, spread to adjacent tissues or both. Seven percent of the patients were reported to be in the distant stage of disease.

This means that almost half of the patients show evidence of regional or systemic disease when first seen.

The Medical Oncologist is confronted with discussing informed consent with this group of patients. His job is not an easy one because the prognosis is guarded and the patient's outcome is predictably poorer.

The options of palliative treatment with radiation and/or chemotherapy have to be adequately discussed in detail with the advanced breast cancer patient. Since these patients with systemic disease are much sicker it is often difficult for the Medical Oncologist to state that the toxic chemotherapeutic agents will have serious side effects. Some effects are: nausea, vomiting, loss of hair, stomatitis, fatigue, etc. and are generally known to the public today. It is difficult for patients to accept this palliative care.

Sometimes, because of the toxic effects of the chemotherapy on the bone marrow (where the red and white cells are made) a suppression of all of the blood elements occurs. Due to a lack of platelets, which are necessary for blood clotting, bleeding can develop and transfusions are necessary. The white cell count can go down and the patient is more prone to get an infection. Antibiotics have to be given and rehospitalization is sometimes necessary. Medicine can be given for the nausea and vomiting and wigs are often worn to cover the loss of hair. Usually the hair grows back once the chemotherapy is stopped. The fatigue and lethargy sometimes leads to depression and those patients often have to be encouraged to continue their chemotherapy.

INFORMED CONSENT AND BREAST RECONSTRUCTION

If the patient has a breast cancer and the treatment recommended is total removal of the breast, reconstruction is discussed. Immediate or delayed reconstruction can be done. If immediate reconstruction is done, either the general surgeon doing the mastectomy or the plastic surgeon can place a silicone implant under the pectoralis major muscle. This is not a difficult procedure. The patient may insist on a plastic surgeon because the remaining breast sometimes has to be made smaller (reduction mammoplasty) and revisions may have to be done at a later date.

Immediate reconstruction is not without its risks and if a major complication develops, the doctor is dealing with a very unhappy patient. That patient is already emotionally drained by the mastectomy and is poorly prepared to withstand the emotional impact of poor reconstruction results such as a slough of a skin flap, infection, or prolonged hospitalization.

Delayed reconstruction is usually recommended unless the patient insists on immediate reconstruction. This allows time for the doctor to watch that patient for local recurrence and also allows the patient to adjust to the absence of the breast.

If delayed reconstruction is done, complete examination of the excised tissue and nodal status to determine extent of disease can be evaluated and this allows for determination of estrogen and progesterone levels quantitatively so that progress may be predicted and if necessary, future treatment planned.

Not all patients qualify for breast reconstruction and they are told this (advanced breast disease with extensive lymph node metastases or diffuse bone or lung metastases, for example).

They are also told that breast reconstruction will not make their body image the same as it was and that the reconstructed breast, whether it be a silicone implant or muscle transfer, may interfere with the doctor's ability to watch the patient's chest wall for recurrent breast cancer.

QUESTION AND ANSWERS

Q. How do you try to inform the patient concerning risks and complications of treatment?

A. A method that can be used is to have the patient come in with the husband or partner (grown children also sometimes) and discuss all options prior to treatment. The secretary can take notes that document the discussion so that no misunderstanding occurs. These notes can be included in the patient's chart.

Q. How do you feel about using long informed consent forms that the patients read and sign prior to treatment?

A. Long legal forms have been devised with numerous questions and answers and there is no such thing as a form that would cover all aspects of breast disease that would include various diagnostic methods, proposed treatment, and all risks and complications that may occur.

Q. Would you elaborate on that?

A. The problem is not to have a long legalistic form for the patient to sign but rather to have a complete definition of treatment that the patient might understand. This is impossible in today's society since we do not have a total accepted answer as to how you should treat the breast cancer patient. There are many alternative methods of treatment.

Q. After the patient has been informed can the patient refuse treatment?

A. Any patient can refuse treatment if they are mentally competent, but this can be a difficult problem for the doctor. I have had patients refuse treatment and then come back three months later and want you to treat them. There's obvious delay in treatment in this type of case and the results are not as good. This type of case has to be well documented.

A percentage of patients will delay, even at risk to themselves and possible spread of their tumor for long periods of time, before accepting treatment.

8

Usual Treatment Methods

In 1775, Patrick Henry made this statement: "I have but one lamp by which my feet are guided and that is the lamp of experience. I know of no way of judging the future but by the past." This statement applies to today's modern treatment of breast cancer.

For nearly a century a diagnosis of breast cancer routinely led to a radical mastectomy, in which surgeons removed the entire breast as well as the lymph nodes in the armpit and underlying chest muscle tissue.

Practically all women died if they developed breast cancer 100 years ago. The disease was not recognized early, surgery was primitive, radiation (x-ray) had not been discovered yet, and there was no such thing as chemotherapy or immunotherapy to help prevent recurrence.

Surgical treatment for cancer of the breast was introduced by Dr. William S. Halsted,[68] a Johns Hopkins surgeon, in the late 19th century. Halsted felt that if you excised the cancer when it was localized to the breast, you could cure the patient. He also felt that cancer of the breast spread to the lymph glands under the armpit (axillary nodes) and that these glands acted as a blockage to further spread of the disease.

If the glands became involved, Halsted's en bloc resection (resection of the breast muscles and glands; i.e. radical mastectomy) would also cure the patient. As the disease involved more extensive numbers of the glands, the cancer would spread throughout the body. Halsted did not believe that cancer of the breast spread via the bloodstream.

This treatment in the early 1900's would have to be considered heroic treatment today, when one considers that there were no antibiotics to give the patient if an infection occurred. Blood transfusions were not being given yet and the anesthesia was primitive, and little or no thoughts were given to cosmetic appearance or reconstruction of the breast. Complications of the surgery did exist and patients were lost at the time of surgery but the survival rate of breast cancer improved.

The operation devised by Halsted became the popular treatment for cancer of the breast and now held out some hope for patients afflicted with the disease. Fifty percent of the patients survived five years. There were also other benefits from this radical surgical approach for treatment of breast cancer. The tissue that was removed allowed the pathologists to study the various types of malignant tumors of the breast and how they behaved. An analysis of the lymph nodes was done and the first attempt at staging disease evolved. (Staging is the process by which doctors learn the extent of the cancer, and how best to treat it. Cancers in Stage I are localized and the most curable. Stage IV are the most advanced and harder to control cases of breast cancer.)

By today's standards, few of the patients of Dr. William S. Halsted would even be operated on because of the size of their tumors. Radiation and chemotherapy would be more practical alternatives.

About the time that Halsted was popularizing radical mastectomy, Wilhelm Conrad Roentgen,[69,70] a German physicist, discovered Roentgen Rays (x-rays) in 1895. Roentgen received the Nobel Prize in medicine for his discovery which allowed the physician to look into the human body and outline its structures (bones, lungs, brain, etc.). Roentgen developed the concept of radiation first for diagnosis and then for therapy in the treatment of cancer.

Many of the breast cancers that Dr. Halsted treated, when first seen, were large primary tumors with obvious or predictable spread. Surgery alone could not hope to cure these women and the long-term results of radical mastectomy were often disappointing. It was not long before radiation therapy was used in follow-up treatment of breast cancer patients.

This combined treatment method: i.e., radical surgery followed by radiation therapy, did not improve survival but did cut down on local recurrence on the chest wall in the fields of radiation therapy treatment.

In the early 1940's a Scotchman by the name of Robert McWhirter[71] began to challenge the need for radical surgery and removal of the muscles in the treatment of breast cancer. He started treating breast cancer with simple mastectomy (removing the breast but not the muscles) followed by radiation. He declared that his method was just as good as Halsted's radical mastectomy.

It was soon recognized that it would be impossible to compare results of his treatment with the radical mastectomy and radiation treatment group, since no tissue (glands) was taken from under the armpit for microscopic study and it would be impossible to determine if you were dealing with local breast cancer or breast cancer with regional nodes involved. In other words, you would be comparing apples and oranges.

In the 1960's and 1970's a growing dissatisfaction with the results of treatment of radical surgical and radical radiotherapy of cancer of the breast developed. It was surmised that the radical surgical treatment of the localized breast cancer and regional nodes whether it be to the armpit (axilla) or to the sternum (internal mammary nodes) or the use of radical radiation therapy to control the disease in the regional lymph nodes had gone as far as it could go. It was decided that controlled trials would have to take place and this was done.

After the trials, researchers[72,73] in different sections of the world arrived at two main conclusions concerning survival. 1) When a patient has radical breast surgery there is no increased survival in giving post-operative radiation therapy and 2) When post-operative radiation therapy is given there is no advantage of a radical mastectomy over a simpler procedure (a simple mastectomy).

What this meant was that radical surgery and radiation therapy had gone as far as it could go in the treatment of cancer of the breast and that some other method would have to be devised to improve survival or some other type of prevention of spread of the cancer would have to be developed.

It was recognized that as a breast cancer grows, eventually, if there is delay in treatment, one is no longer dealing with a localized problem and as the tumor gets large enough, spread of the cancer occurs and one is now dealing with a diffuse disseminated systemic disease (either thru lymphatics or blood stream). As to when this dissemination occurs still is debated since the exact methods by which an individual patient handles free cancer cells (immune mechanism) is still not determined.

In other words, if you have a small tumor which is detected early, it can still be localized and the results of treatment are good (either by surgery or radiation). However, if the tumor is bigger than 5 cm. when first seen, the incidence of spread of the tumor is over fifty percent and now you are dealing with a more difficult systemic problem to solve.

In 1971, the National Cancer Institute started an in-depth clinical study to see if lesser radical procedures were comparable to radical mastectomy. Three types of treatment methods were compared: 1) radical mastectomy, 2) simple mastectomy (breast removal only), and 3) total mastectomy followed by radiation therapy. The results showed no difference in patient survival.

This study has led most surgeons to do some form of modified mastectomy in the treatment of breast cancer. In most major centers a total mastectomy (removal of all breast tissue plus the removal of sufficient nodes under the armpit (axilla) to stage the disease is recognized as the current standard treatment for most breast cancers. (See Figure 5)

Today, it has been shown that radiation therapy has done little to increase survival after good surgery and most Oncologists base their treatment on the stage of the disease and whether the glands are involved with cancer or not.

Bonadonna and his associates[74] at the National Tumor Cancer Institute in Milan, Italy, in 1976, reported on combination chemotherapy as an adjuvant treatment in operable breast cancer.

They reported improved survival rates and a reduction in the local recurrence rates in the pre-menopausal group of women with breast cancer who received triple chemotherapy. At the present time, if more than three glands in the axilla are involved with cancer, chemotherapy is recommended.

The rationale for giving chemotherapy if more than three lymph glands are involved with breast cancer is that one is now dealing with systemic disease and since surgery and radiation treatment has gone as far as it can go, perhaps drugs can kill the free floating cancer cells and improve survival rates in the advanced cancer.

MODIFIED MASTECTOMY AND AXILLARY DISSECTION

The operation done most frequently today is the removal of the breast tissue and a sampling of the glands in the armpit (axilla) to stage the disease.

Most breast cancer surgeons have been reluctant to accept the concept of lumpectomy or lumpectomy and radiation therapy for breast cancer

Figure 5

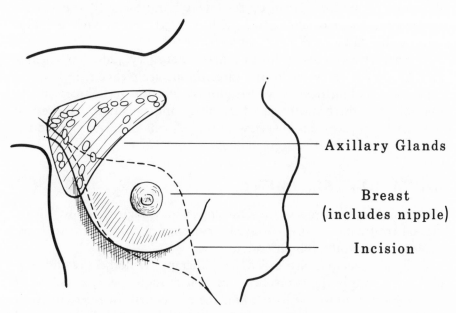

Axillary Glands

Breast
(includes nipple)

Incision

MODIFIED MASTECTOMY
AND AXILLARY DISSECTION

Removal of Entire Breast and
Axillary Lymphnodes – Leaving
chest muscles intact. (Transverse
Incision can be used also.)

patients because they do not wish to abandon a well proven method of treatment that has been in existence for many years. Stage I cancers of the breast treated by mastectomy and axillary dissection have an eighty percent survival rate and it is difficult to visualize how those results can be improved.

Plastic surgical techniques have also improved immensely and the immediate or delayed reconstruction of the breast with a silicone gel prosthesis has helped reduce the psychic trauma associated with the loss of the breast. Breast cancer surgeons feel that by doing a mastectomy, the risk of leaving cancer behind in another segment of the breast (multicentric breast cancer) is reduced since a wider excision around the tumor is accomplished. Some cancer specialists feel that to remove the entire breast for a small cancer (Stage I and Stage II) is excessive surgery and lesser or alternative methods of treatment such as lumpectomy should be used (see Chapter 9).

The main treatments for breast cancer are surgery, radiation, chemotherapy, or combinations of the three. None are pleasant, but we are constantly finding new ways to improve surgical techniques and to minimize the discomfort caused by drugs and radiation. The rest of this chapter presents an overview of these forms of treatment and the side effects that most concern women.

RADIATION TREATMENT

Sometimes, after surgery, the Oncologist may suggest follow-up radiation treatments to prevent local recurrence or to treat microscopic foci of cancer in the lymph nodes.

Radiation therapy, also called x-ray therapy, radiotherapy and irradiation, is simply the controlled emission of high-energy rays. When used against a tumor, radiation kills the cancer cells or interferes with their ability to reproduce, and the tumor shrinks in size. With external radiation, different units are used with different energy sources. The type of machine and the radiation dosage will depend upon the size and location of the tumor, as well as the availability of the devices. Smaller hospitals may have just one unit.

Because radiation treatment is so specialized a field, it is important that anyone receiving such treatment has it administered by a person trained and certified in therapeutic radiation (as opposed to diagnostic radiation). The person will be thoroughly experienced in knowing what dosages to give and how to give the maximum dosage to breast tumors with minimal damage to normal cells.

Should radiation treatments be necessary, you will meet with a radiotherapist before receiving treatment. At this time you might undergo x-rays to determine the exact size of the tumor and its location. Nuclear magnetic resonance machines are also being used for this purpose. Then the tumor's position will be marked with a tatoo (ink) so the radiotherapist will know exactly where to direct the radiation. The number of treatments will vary depending upon the tumor. Usually they will be given over a period of four to five weeks, typically in many short sessions.

Not surprisingly, people are nervous about radiation treatment. Many stories about the side effects harken back to the old days of radiation burns and severe nausea. Today, even with newer and safer units, women still worry. The most common question is: "Will it hurt?" The answer to this is no. However, you can expect some side effects, perhaps including a sunburned look and a roughness in the area being treated. These may not appear until the fourth or fifth day after treatment begins or possibly later. Other side effects and suggestions about self-care are included in a booklet available from the National Cancer Institute called "Radiation Therapy and You" (Appendix E).

If you have a small tumor which is detected early, it can be localized and successfully treated with radiation or surgery. However, if the tumor is larger than one and one-half inch when first seen, there is a fifty percent chance it has spread to the lymph nodes or other parts of the body. In such cases, simple excision of a lump in the breast will leave cancer cells behind in at least twenty-five percent of patients.[75]

To eradicate the malignancy and prevent it from recurring, a high dose of radiation (5000-6500 rads) has to be given to the breast and suspicious nodes in the armpit. This dose is sometimes enhanced by needle implants under general anesthesia and the cost is comparable to surgical treatment.

As with mastectomy, there is disagreement over the benefits and risks of radiation therapy for breast cancer. Several studies indicate that high-dosage radiation affects the body's immune system, increasing the chance of breast cancer spreading to other parts of the body.[76,77] There is also the long-term effects of prolonged radiation for which few clinical studies exist, and the swelling or edema that occurs in the arm when radiation therapy is used.

Not everyone can or should have radiation treatment for breast cancer. It is, however, an accepted method that is finding many adherents in this country and throughout the world. In France, for example, the treatment of choice is lumpectomy followed by radiation therapy. Every woman should have this option discussed with her as well as types of surgery and chemotherapy now available.

CHEMOTHERAPY

Chemotherapy is the use of drugs for the treatment and control of disease. While any disease can be treated this way, the term today usually refers to cancer treatment. The aim is either to completely destroy the cancer cells or in some way to interfere with their ability to reproduce. It is believed that anti-cancer drugs alter the cancer cell's ability to divide and survive.

Different families of drugs are used in chemotherapy. Some are highly toxic alkylating agents that short-circuit messages directing cell division (Ex. cytoxan). Some are antimetabolites which kill cancer cells by mimicking substances required for cell growth (methotrexate, fluorouracil). Some are extracts of plants which act as antibiotics to disrupt the myriad functions of cancer cells (actinomycin, mitomycin). A fourth category of anticancer drugs are also used which inhibit construction of proteins vital to cell division (vinblastine, vincristine).

Because the side effects of these drugs can be serious, the physician must maintain a delicate balance between dose and frequency by giving enough chemotherapy to kill cancer cells without permanently destroying too many normal tissues. Individuals also tolerate drugs differently, so any unexplained event should be reported to your doctor immediately. When treatment is stopped, most side effects disappear including anemia or hair loss. To cope with the loss of appetite, common among patients receiving chemotherapy (and radiation treatment), guidelines and food tips are available in a booklet "Nutrition for the Cancer Patient" that can be obtained from the U.S. Department of Health and Human Services (Appendix E).

Rapidly growing cancer cells are most vulnerable to chemotherapy. The drugs used produce more injury to cancer cells than to normal cells. There is a disagreement as to whether chemotherapy should be used in cases of breast cancer where the disease has not spread. In fact, it is discouraged by the National Institutes of Health (NIH) which reports that mastectomy alone gives an eighty percent survival rate. Wouldn't chemotherapy help the other twenty percent? Possibly, but to give everyone chemotherapy as a matter of routine means that too many women would receive too much toxicity in more cases than will be useful. Again, this is a question about which you should seek individual advice.

Chemotherapy also suppresses the immune system. A serious side effect is the suppression of the bone marrow, which is vital to the production of white and red blood cells. Anticancer drugs, like radiation, also can severely impair the system and cause new cancers in some patients. There is substantial evidence that certain drugs affect the liver and kidneys, further limiting the body's natural response to diseases including cancer. To protect against serious side effects, your physician can perform special blood tests to determine how anticancer drugs are affecting you.

Most chemotherapy is given on an outpatient basis in the doctor's office or hospital. However, for some patients short periods of hospitalization may be necessary to monitor treatment. Before chemotherapy begins, the physician should explain the reactions that might occur during the administration of specific drugs. You should ask for any available "Patient Medication Instructions." Information about one hundred drugs is now available in easy-to-read leaflets put out by the American Medical Association and distributed free through doctors.

OTHER FORMS OF TREATMENT

In addition to radiation and chemotherapy, several newer forms of treatment are being tried in patients with cancer of the breast. Some, like lipid vesicles, are still very much in the experimental stage. Others, including hormonal manipulation, are important therapies in the management of patients with breast cancer. The principal new treatments are:

Hormone Therapies Hormonal therapy may provide prolonged control in many patients with breast cancer. This is why, whenever a breast biopsy is done and a cancer is detected, the tissue should be analyzed for estrogen and progesterone binding. Shrinkage or disappearance of the cancer may occur and the cancer may go into remission for long periods of time. In fact, the National Institutes of Health has recently endorsed hormonal therapy with the drug tamoxifen as a "treatment of choice" for many older women with regional spread of the disease. (Tamoxifen is a hormone-blocking drug which induces a sort of chemical oophorectomy and is not recommended in women of child-bearing age.)

Immunotherapy Several methods are being used, all of which show some promise in the treatment of breast cancer. One uses chemically-altered tumor cells to stimulate an anticancer response from the body. Another uses antibodies harvested from one person to fight cancer in another. A third method involves the injection of substances that may trigger natural anticancer mechanisms.

Hyperthermia Not entirely new (induced high fever was used to treat cancer patients sixty years ago), computer-controlled hyperthermia uses heat-producing energy to selectively attack cancer cells. In tests on patients who have failed to respond to conventional therapy, researchers have found hyperthermia treatment, when combined with radiation therapy, can be twice as effective as radiation alone. Immersing the patient in hot water baths also appears to increase the effectiveness of chemotherapy and radiation according to the National Cancer Institute.

Lipid Vesicles These are microscopic fatty capsules used to deliver anticancer drugs directly to the tumor, thereby reducing harmful side effects by bypassing other tissues. Injected into the bloodstream, the vesicles release the drug at just the right place to be most effective. Another method uses antigens to activate the immune response of normal cells—putting them on guard as the vesicle passes by en route to the tumor site.

Interferon Possibly the most important agent in stimulating the body's immune system, interferon has been shown to stop the spread of cancer in animal experiments, but publicity is far ahead of its known usefulness in the treatment of breast cancer. The high cost and short supply of the substances have also hindered research until recently.

Photoradiation For this experimental treatment, a patient is given a photoactive material intravenously. The material accumulates in the tumor area and surrounding tissues, where it can be activated by a laser beam to destroy the cancer cells. Other new methods of treating breast cancer may be available for some patients. Ask your physician whether such a program exists in your area and whether you qualify.

SUMMARY

In spite of what you read in newspapers and magazines and hear about on television and radio, the most common operation used in the treatment of breast cancer today is a removal of the breast (modified mastectomy) and a sampling of the glands in the armpit (axillary dissection) to stage the disease (70% of the cases). (See Figure 5) Unfortunately, almost fifty percent of breast cancer patients first present in an advanced stage of the disease (Stage III or Stage IV) and do not qualify for breast conservation surgery, such as lumpectomy.

With the new imaging devices (mammography, xeromammography, ultrasound) more and more minimal breast cancers are being detected before a woman can feel the lump. How you treat this type of breast cancer and the controversies related to this treatment are discussed in the next chapter (9).

9

Limited Surgery; Does It Work?

"Limited surgery works as well as removal of the entire breast for women with breast cancer in the earlier stages" (Stage I and Stage II). This statement may be true and definitely gives hope to all women who are fortunate enough to be diagnosed with a small breast cancer. We are now detecting cancers that you can not feel. With sophisticated imaging devices such as mammography, xeromammography, and ultrasound we are finding breast cancers earlier. This means that the breast cancer specialists are now treating a new group of patients that they never saw before, since prior to development of the imaging devices, almost all breast cancers were detected by breast self-examination by the patient (80%), and the cancers that could be felt were larger and more advanced.

The technique of limited surgery removes only the breast lump with the tumor and adjacent tissue around the cancer to obtain margins which are then studied. In addition to the partial surgery on the breast, a sampling of the glands under the armpit is done to see if the cancer has spread to the lymph nodes (axillary dissection). (See Figure 6) This allows for proper staging of the disease and helps determine whether the woman will need radiation therapy to treat disease in the glands and may also need some form of chemotherapy to try to destroy any cancer cells that may be in the body's systemic circuit.

Figure 6

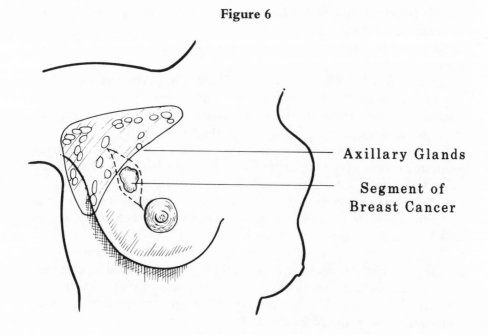

Axillary Glands

Segment of
Breast Cancer

SEGMENTECTOMY (Lumpectomy) AND AXILLARY GLAND REMOVAL

- Preserves Breast Contour.
- Radiation Therapy given after Surgery.

Radiation therapy is given to the breast after the lumpectomy is done to cut down on local recurrence and to attempt to destroy any other possible foci of cancer that may be developing (multicentric cancer).

This recent research from the National Surgical Adjuvant Breast Project[78] proposes that limited surgery (segmentectomy) does work on small breast tumors less than 4 cms. in size. More and more breast conservation operations will probably be done in selected cases in the future.

Unfortunately, not every woman with a breast cancer qualifies for breast conservation surgery and this is the hardest part for a woman to accept. Almost fifty percent of women, when first seen with breast cancer, present with a tumor that has already spread to the lymph glands or other parts of her body. In many cases mastectomy may be more appropriate treatment.

Each case has to be individualized prior to treatment. Not all breast cancers are the same size or have the same stage of the disease. The woman's age when she develops the cancer is important as well as the size of her breast. There are also many other variables that have to be considered. Since there are so many different breast care options now, there is mass confusion as to which method is the best.

Limited surgery *does not work* if the woman presents with a large neglected cancer of the breast similar to the type that Halsted took care of many years ago with his radical methods of treatment.

Halsted may be criticized today, but in his day, he made a great contribution in the treatment of breast cancer and he saved many women's lives which would have been lost.

We are now in a transition period from the supraradical operations, to the modified mastectomy, to the breast conservation operations, such as lumpectomy and axillary node sampling to stage the disease. The scientific community is assessing and comparing the new methods of treatment with the older methods.

Breast cancer is one of the most common malignancies in women, and one that deserves the best treatment possible. There is no one approach suited to the needs of all patients. The decision regarding the extent of the surgical procedure, the use of radiation or any other treatment should be based upon extensive diagnostic studies, the kind of cancer reported by the pathologist, the age and preference of the patient and the considered judgment of the cancer surgeon.

The choice of treatment then is one the patient should fully understand. There are now a variety of telephone medical services, approved by medical societies and hospitals, that provide expert and confidential advice on medical problems including cancer. The best of these for the woman with breast cancer is Cancer Hotline (800-638-6694), which was begun by the National Cancer Institute. Another is the Second Opinion Hotline (800-638-6833) which offers phone numbers of clinics and specialists for those who want a second opinion before deciding on surgery.

To help women make an informed choice about breast cancer treatment, the rest of this chapter summarizes the different types of limited surgery and tells how they differ from modified or radical mastectomy. A discussion of the controversies is presented in a question and answer dialogue at the end. All women are encouraged to discuss with their physicians the options available, the details of the recommended approach and the reasons for a specific procedure.

LUMPECTOMY

The term "lumpectomy" is not a good one. It is essentially a biopsy of the tissue to see if a cancer is present. The term can be interpreted in many ways depending upon the philosophy of the operating surgeon. It can be a simple excision of the tumor or a wide extensive excision that has a deforming effect on the breast. The placement of the incision is very important if further surgery is to be contemplated or plastic reconstruction is anticipated.

Women who are very thin or who have small breasts often are unhappy with the results of a lumpectomy. It is also not very successful if the tumor is under the nipple or deep within the breast tissue. When a lumpectomy is done, usually a separate incision has to be made to sample the glands in the armpit for staging purposes.

SEGMENTECTOMY

A segmentectomy is usually a wider excision than a lumpectomy. It often includes the fascia (muscle covering) of the chest muscle. Four or five samples of tissue around the breast cancer are taken to be sure that adequate margins are obtained. Since the majority of breast cancers are in the outer quadrants of the breast, a single incision can often be used so that a sampling of the glands can also be done and a good cosmetic effect can be obtained. (See Figure 6)

The advantages of a lumpectomy or segmental resection are that the breast is normally left intact. In fact, in some sections of the country, no further treatment is given except that the glands under the armpit may be sampled to see if they are free of spread. Because of the high local recurrence rate,[79,80] most centers give post-operative radiation if a lumpectomy or segmentectomy is done.

AXILLARY DISSECTION (Sampling of the glands)

It is recommended that a sampling of the glands be done in almost all cases of breast cancer in order to stage the disease. The cancer surgeon is trying to determine if the disease is localized to the breast or has spread to the glands. The treatment is different if the tumor has metastasized and is in the glands. I personally feel that a complete axillary dissection should be done in all cases because so much depends upon whether the glands are involved or not. Upper levels of lymph glands can be involved[81] and if only a sampling is done, cancer can be missed and the best treatment is not being given.

SUMMARY/QUESTIONS

There is currently a debate over the type of surgery that should be performed on women with breast cancer that may be nearing resolution. In the meantime, modified mastectomy has replaced the more disfiguring radical mastectomy as the treatment of choice. In recent trials lumpectomy and segmentectomy have shown to be effective in the early stages of breast cancer if the treatment is followed by radiation therapy (5000 rads). However, not enough time has elapsed to determine long term results. Initial reports are encouraging.

Q. I should think all women with breast cancer would want to preserve their breast and have a lumpectomy or segmentectomy done rather than having the breast removed (mastectomy).

A. Unfortunately, not all patients qualify for breast conservation surgery. Almost fifty percent have large tumors, evidence of regional spread (lymph glands) or systemic spread (lung, bone, liver, etc.) when first seen.

Q. What does this mean?

A. It means that almost one half of the patients have had a delay in diagnosis and the tumors are larger or may be multicentric (more than one area of the breast involved), and the tumor involves the lymph glands or other organs. Usually a more extensive procedure has to be done (mastectomy and axillary dissection). Radiation therapy and chemotherapy may have to be used to prevent recurrence and increase survival time. In some cases the patient presents with systemic spread and only a biopsy is done to confirm the tissue diagnosis and then palliative treatment is started.

Q. Should women seek a second opinion before surgery for breast cancer?

A. Yes, particularly if she does not have confidence in the doctor recommending her treatment. There is still disagreement over which type of surgery is best for each type of tumor. Each case has to be individualized. However, delaying any surgery for long periods of time is not recommended.

Q. *Who should you see?*

A. You should pick your own cancer specialist for the second opinion. In some cases, you may have to go outside your local community to get the best advice.

Q. *Since there are so many different choices of treatment for the breast cancer patient, how does the patient decide what should be done?*

A. The patient should become better informed and ask questions. She should have confidence in the doctor taking care of her and should be able to communicate well with that individual. She should ask what the size of the tumor is and whether it is localized or not. In some cases she will not have a choice in treatment but she can still refuse. If she has a minimal cancer that is detected by the new imaging devices, she will have a better prognosis and may qualify for the different methods of conservation surgery.

Q. *How many women with breast cancer have limited surgery?*

A. Approximately ten percent in this country, although the number is increasing. In France limited surgery followed by radiation therapy is particularly common. The European countries seem to be ahead of us in the use of limited surgery.

Q. *Why are surgeons still doing modified mastectomies for small cancers?*

A. Surgeons are unwilling to give up a proven operation that produces an eighty percent five year survival rate in Stage I cancers.

Q. *Are there other reasons?*

A. Yes, they argue that breast cancer is not a systemic disease from its onset and if treated properly in the beginning, the woman can be cured by adequate surgery. They feel that the breast with cancer in it will have other separate foci of cancer developing within it (multicentric disease). This is why they argue that the entire breast has to be removed. Since it takes two to eight years for a cancer to grow to a size that you can feel and detect, it will take fifteen to twenty years to determine if simpler treatment methods will produce similar long term survival rates.

Q. *Is there any research to substantiate this?*

A. Yes, a study done by Gallager and Martin[82] confirmed that human breast cancer is not a local process but a disease which affects the breast diffusely in many different areas. Multiple invasive nodules were present in more than forty-five percent of the cases.

Q. *Does the size of the tumor determine the multiple areas of involvement of the breast?*

A. Yes, many cancer centers[83,84] have found that the likelihood of finding cancer in more than one area of the breast is related to the primary tumor size. What this means is that a minimal cancer (smaller than 5 mm. in size) in all likelihood does not have other cancers growing in the breast. Whereas a breast cancer that you can feel is more likely to have other sites of cancer developing. Studies have been done that show that breast cancers larger than two inches have a fifty percent chance of having spread to other areas of the body.

Q. *What do the breast conservation experts and radiation therapists have to say about this?*

A. They argue that radiation therapy can control the primary site after the tumor has been removed and destroy the multicentric areas of cancer which may be left behind or within the regional lymphatics. Some argue that the microscopic foci of cancer left behind can be handled by the host's immune mechanism and the small cancer will not progress to actual disease.

Q. *Why was radiation therapy added to lumpectomy?*

A. Because in previous studies[85] in which lumpectomy alone was done, there was a high incidence of local recurrence. It was felt that radiation would prevent local recurrence and increase survival. Radiation is also given if the glands are positive. Chemotherapy is also added.

Q. *Why do radiation therapists think that radiation will work following lumpectomy when radiation therapy did not increase survival following radical mastectomy?*

A. They feel that a higher dose of radiation is now being given (5000 rads) and boosting doses of 1500 rads to the local site. They also feel that the newer machines with computers do a better job.

Q. *Are there some breast cancers that can be removed by lumpectomy without any further treatment?*

A. Yes, carcinoma in situ or lobular carcinoma in situ of the breast, since it may take twenty years before invasive carcinoma develops. New imaging devices should be able to pick up changes of invasion and proper treatment given.

Q. *Does age play a role in the choice of treatment for the woman with a small breast cancer (less than 1¹/₂ inches)?*

A. I feel it does. If the woman chooses a lumpectomy followed by radiation therapy and is 55–65 years old, I don't worry as much about delayed adverse radiation changes that may develop. It takes 15–20 years for a radiation induced cancer to show up. If the woman is young (35 years of age) I do worry about it.

Q. *Are there any other adverse reactions to radiation?*

A. Yes, you get changes to the skin from radiation and fibrotic changes in the remaining breast tissue. Also tissues do not heal as well after radiation therapy. It's also more difficult to follow these patients. The immune system is affected by radiation with a suppression and some cancer specialists feel that when this occurs you're more apt to get metastatic disease.

Q. *Does radiation therapy after lumpectomy change the method of follow-up for the patient?*

A. Yes, because radiation therapy produces a hardness and a fibrotic feel to the breast. It can also cause calcific changes suggestive of recurrence. It means that more frequent mammograms and sometimes more needle biopsies have to be done. Ultrasound is also being used as an aid to detect recurrence.

Q. *Should more surgeons be doing more segmentectomies (limited surgery) for breast cancer?*

A. Only a selected group of women with small tumors qualify for breast conservation surgery followed by radiation treatment. However, since similar results as mastectomy are being projected more women will probably take the chance to preserve their breast. New x-ray treatment techniques are providing better local, regional control. I feel that limited surgery can be done successfully for small breast cancers. There is a worry about the larger breast cancers (4 cm in size) being treated successfully by limited surgery and radiation, since the size of tumor determines the amount of other area breast involvement and incidence of regional or systemic spread. (See Figure 4)

10

Cancer and the Foods You Eat

You are what you eat. Every person does not eat the same food. Women particularly are conscious of the foods they eat and their personal appearance is very important to them. Dieting is part of their daily regimen.

As a woman gets older and approaches the menopause, there is a tendency to put on weight and attitudes may change. If she becomes frustrated or unhappy with her lifestyle, she may use eating as a method to relieve that frustration. Don't do it! That fudge, peanut butter and particularly excessive animal fat consumption will do you in. The lifestyle of today with fast food consumption, if done in excess, will increase your cholesterol levels and triglycerides so that not only will you be at increased risk for heart attacks but cancer also.

As a woman approaches menopause, her hormones change, her exercise pattern may decrease, and the middle age spread can become noticeable and alarming. She should reassess what is happening and decide to watch her diet, maintain a daily exercise regimen and try to prevent the problems of obesity.

There are many risk factors considered to be important that may cause breast cancer. Diet has been suspected as a major cause.[86] The link between nutrition and breast cancer in particular is very strong and our tendency to consume fatty foods at a young age, which is increasing, may be extremely hazardous in the future. In countries like Japan, where fatty meat is not the main source of protein, breast cancer rates drop significantly.[87,88,89] By contrast, the fat intake per day in the United States is three to four times that of the Japanese. In Japan the total fat consumption in the diet is low. More fish and staples, other than beef, are eaten. The risk of getting breast cancer in Japan is significantly lower.

Increased dietary fat intake causing obesity, increases the insulin requirement in the human body to maintain sugar metabolic equilibrium and probably causes the body's estrogen levels to increase which places the female at greater risk to getting breast cancer.

Japanese women have much lower levels of estrogen than Americans. When Japanese women, however, move to this country and change their lifestyle, their consumption of dietary fat increases and the incidence of breast cancer increases also, approaching the level of other American women.[90]

I asked all of my breast cancer patients about their dietary habits and weight. Over fifty percent were overweight and admitted to trying to lose weight by trying unusual dietary methods. The overweight women with breast cancer admitted that they liked specific foods. Steak, beef, and hamburger were mentioned most often (more than 45%) suggesting that high beef consumption, which often has a higher concentration of triglycerides, may be a factor in the development of breast cancer.

The socioeconomic factors associated with breast cancer are quite obvious. One must be able to afford the cost of a diet rich in fats and cholesterol (beef, milk, protein, etc.)—a typical diet in the U.S.A. and Europe.

There are numerous theories to explain why a high fat diet is unhealthy and why obese women are more inclined to develop cancer of the breast and uterus than lean women. Perhaps such foods promote the secretion in the breast of the hormone prolactin, or carry possible carcinogens that feed cancer cells, or modify the body's immune mechanisms so that we cannot defend ourselves against breast cancer. Perhaps fat itself is cancer-causing.

Whatever the reasons we cannot escape the fact that nutrition or the lack of it is a principal risk factor in the development of breast cancer. Recently nutritionists have suggested that the consumption of certain foods help prevent cancer. For instance, people who eat cabbage frequently have less cancer than people who don't. Cabbage and other cruciferous vegetables, such as broccoli and brussel sprouts are considered good sources of fiber and vitamins. It is not known which components in these vegetables help prevent cancer.

It has also been found that foods rich in beta-carotene, which the body converts to vitamin A, are associated with lower risks of cancers of all kinds. Those foods include apricots, peaches, citrus fruits, and deep yellow vegetables, such as carrots, yellow turnips, and winter squash.

Diet, Nutrition and Cancer published by the National Academy Press in 1982[91] is an excellent reference for those individuals wanting an in depth study of the role of diet and nutrition in cancer. This can be obtained from U.S. Government Services.

Before storming the supermarket for cabbage, carrots or other foods that might prevent cancer, it's important to understand what is meant by good nutrition—and how it relates to women and breast cancer. For one thing, not all foods are as good as we think they are, and other supposedly "natural" foods may contain more additives and calories than we would suspect.

The important thing is to exercise prudence and common sense about what you eat—try taking in less calories and less fats. Each day eat some whole-grain cereals, fruits and vegetables, particularly those high in vitamin C and beta-carotene. Cut down on your intake of pickled and smoked foods like sausages, and bacon or hot dogs. Avoid too much alcohol, particularly if you smoke cigarettes. It boosts the risk of cancer in those women not otherwise at risk.

Whether or not you should add vitamin supplements to your diet to prevent cancer is a matter of controversy. While all of the claims cannot be proved, few will argue that a woman adding vitamins to a balanced diet low in fats will probably feel healthier and be healthier. She may also be reducing her cancer risk. This was first demonstrated by Dr. Linus Pauling[92] a decade ago in his studies of vitamin C and cancer prevention, and in studies of other vitamins since then.

Research has shown that specific vitamins, whether in the foods we eat or as tablets, can inhibit the growth of cancer cells and help in the healing of precancerous lesions.[93,94] There is little evidence, however, that massive doses of these same vitamins can be more effective in treating patients with advanced stages of cancer. For example, in my study of breast cancer patients, forty-six percent said they took vitamin

C daily or one of the multivitamin supplements. One-third reported that they took vitamin E.

CAFFEINE AND ADDITIVES

Not everything we eat causes cancer. Caffeine, for example, has been linked to fibrocystic disease[95,96] which some believe to be a precursor to cancer. However, there is little evidence to support such findings and other types of benign breast disease may have a more malignant potential (hyperplasia, papillomotosis).

The caffeine in coffee, tea, and cola drinks is harmful to people with a heart condition or peptic ulcers because it increases the flow of blood to the heart and the amount of acid and pepsin in the stomach. It is also a lipolytic agent which helps to break down fats and in this way can lead to an increase in your weight. Caffeine may also cause birth defects if pregnant women drink it in substantial amounts. Gradually try to limit your intake. Don't go cold turkey—that can disrupt the body's cycle and cause headaches. Instead get yourself down to a cup a day.

People have become so concerned about the bad things in foods, it might be reassuring to know there are many that are good for you. Sweet acidophilus milk, for example, may prevent breast cancer. Tests of this low-fat milk indicate that it helps lower the levels of enzymes responsible for generating carcinogens and may limit circulation of estrogen and cholesterol, both suspected cancer-causting agents. There's more than a grain of truth to fiber diet claims, mainly because chewy fiber foods take longer to eat and create a feeling of fullness, thereby aiding in weight control.

Food additives are another story. They have little or no nutritive value and some are actually suspected carcinogens. In addition, only a small proportion of these substances are tested to see if they do cause cancer. They are used to make food look better (red dye in beef), taste better (saccharin, caramel), or stay fresh longer. The only way you can be sure foods are "natural" is to buy fresh fruits, vegetables, meats, dairy products, and fish exclusively.

A list of ingredients is mandatory on most foods, but the words can mean whatever the manufacturer wants. According to the U.S. Department of Agriculture, many foods advertised as "natural" contain additives, preservatives, artificial coloring or other ingredients. The evidence against unsaturated fatty acids such as those in sunflower oil may be just as incriminating as against saturated fats such as butter and lard. Check food labels for all ingredients and suspicious additives, as well as number of calories, vitamin and mineral content.

Studies have shown that as our bodies age we become much more susceptible to the harmful effects of food additives, fatty foods and improper diet. This is especially true for the woman at the menopause who is more at risk of developing breast cancer. Keeping weight down and getting enough vitamins are doubly important at this often stressful time in one's life.

STRESS AND ALCOHOL

Stress can play a role in the etiology of breast cancer as it is known to do in other diseases. Certain foods are known to increase or decrease stress in the same way that they cause allergies. This research on diet behavior suggests that what we eat can affect our moods by altering certain brain chemicals or neurotransmitters. Even skeptics agree that people who are well nourished tend to feel better and have more energy. Clearly, if you want to take care of your mental health, you can't ignore your diet.

The best eating plan for mental—and physical—health will contain fresh, unprocessed foods. You should limit consumption of animal protein because of its high fat content. Emphasize vegetables, fruits, whole grains, and nuts. These foods are the best sources of mood-stabilizing vitamins and minerals such as magnesium, calcium and the B vitamins. They also give off sugar slowly and, consequently, help keep energy and temper even. Fresh salt water fish is an excellent source of protein without high fat content.

Drinking too much alcohol can also be bad if you want to stay on an even keel. Alcohol stimulates the body's production of insulin, causing effects on blood sugar, energy and mood similar to those produced by eating processed foods. A hospital study has shown a definite link between alcohol and breast cancer in patients who were heavy drinkers.[97]

Some of the reasons why alcohol puts women at risk to develop breast cancer are known while others are only now being investigated.[98] For one thing, alcoholic drinks are high in calories which can lead to obesity and liver damage. The latter, as we know, is the body's enzyme-producing factory and a vital part of defense mechanisms against cancer.

Alcoholic drinks also contain nitrosamines, additives and preservatives which are known or suspected carcinogens. So much so that the World Health Organization[99] has seen fit to label excessive consumption of alcoholic beverages as a causative factor in many types of cancer. The body is only able to metabolize about one ounce of whiskey in an hour so that several drinks at one time causes a marked increase in alcohol blood concentration with all of the obvious toxic effects.

No one alcoholic beverage is better than another, either. Beer drinkers are just as apt to develop cancer as those who favor gin or scotch. Mixed drinks are no less toxic than whiskey "on the rocks." It is the total alcoholic content and not the type of beverage that causes the damage—and the best advice is to drink in moderation or not at all. This is particularly true for pregnant women since as little as an ounce a day of alcohol can lead to a significant decrease in a baby's weight at birth, and increase the likelihood of spontaneous abortion.

If you're interested in finding out what your favorite libation includes (few companies freely disclose what they put into their products), a booklet "Chemical Additives in Booze" can be obtained from the Center for Science in the Public Interest (Appendix E). The organization has been trying since 1972 to get the federal government to require the listing of ingredients on alcoholic beverages.

DIET AND EXERCISE

You should, of course, exercise regularly to get all of the benefits of a proper diet. There may be individual aspects—for example, high blood pressure, cardiac disease, chronic lung problems—that rule out some forms of exercise. Your previous medical history may also limit your athletic schedule. The odds are that your doctor won't raise any barriers to your exercising.

Research shows that such a program can also help your body to cope better with stress, and can contribute to a speedier recovery from everyday infections. The body is an efficient factory for the disposal of all sorts of harmful chemicals if the organs are functioning properly. Muscles, heart, and lungs all depend on food and exercise to work efficiently and to eliminate waste products. Bone marrow and lymph tissue, in particular, play an important part in cancer prevention.

The lymph glands, which are in many parts of your body, act as a filtering system to resist infection or disease and are a source of lymphocytes (white blood cells) which produce cancer antibodies. Lymph passes through a series of filters or nodes and is ultimately returned to the bloodstream.

All that a healthy person needs to do for lymph, blood and bone marrow is to maintain an adequate diet, avoid toxic substances and exercise to keep the body healthy and prevent infections. Something else to remember is that while one in thirteen women develop breast cancer, twelve do not. Something is protecting them, and part of that something could be in the foods they eat and their lifestyle.

SUMMARY/QUESTIONS

Experts tell us that the cause of some cancers may be what we eat. How can you find out what food in particular is the cause—and what foods should you eat? The best tactic is to be your own cancer detective. Read food labels for calories, additives and other ingredients. Purchase fresh vegetables, fruits, meats and fish whenever you can. Avoid alcohol in great quantities so that your body is better able to function as an immune system. Even more important, avoid becoming overweight and get lots of exercise.

Q. *Why all the publicity about vitamin E?*

A. Several studies showed that vitamin E helped to relieve the pain associated with fibrocystic breast disease. However, the antioxidant properties of this substance (tocopherol) does not work in all patients and it is already fairly widely distributed in any balanced diet.

Q. *Does vitamin E have other effects on the body?*

A. Vitamin E has been called the fertility vitamin and some women have felt that their ovarian function has been stimulated by the use of this vitamin.

Q. *What about megadoses of vitamins?*

A. Massive doses of any vitamin or mineral can create a toxic overload. Some of the possible effects are headaches, blurred vision, and impaired hormonal action and blood circulation.[100,101] If a dose is large enough, vitamins stop acting like foods and start acting like drugs.

Q. *Are some vitamins better than others?*

A. It depends. The vitamins to especially look out for are A, D, and E. They are not water soluble, and so are not excreted daily in urine.

Instead they build up in the body and an overdose can be harmful.

Q. *What minerals help to prevent breast cancer?*

A. Potassium for one—invisible, tasteless, but vital. When we lower our sodium intake while increasing potassium, blood pressure is reduced because potassium discourages the body from retaining water. Calcium and magnesium also help in blood circulation and bone marrow production. Good sources of all three are bananas, chicken, cantaloupes, skim milk, yogurt, and green leafy vegetables.

Q. *You seem not to mention beef—is there a reason?*

A. Yes. Beef is a major source of unsaturated fats and grilling generates small amounts of carcinogens. The evidence from countries who consume far less beef than we do is just too hard to ignore.

Q. *Is the food in fast food restaurants good for you?*

A. Most of the food in fast food restaurants is fried: hamburgers, french fries, chicken, etc. and contains a lot of fats and calories. There may be high amounts of sodium and saturated fats used in the cooking also. Moderation should prevail in eating these foods.

Q. *What should we eat instead of beef?*

A. More fish, chicken, and fresh vegetables—especially those high in B and C vitamins. A deficiency of vitamin B affects nearly all the body tissues, particularly those containing rapidly dividing cells. Vitamin C helps maintain healthy tissue and the integrity of cell walls.

Q. *Why do you seem to play down cholesterol?*

A. It's not the cholesterol content but the total amount of fat in the diet that contributes to breast cancer. This leads to increased free fatty acid levels (triglycerides) which impair the body's immune mechanisms.

Q. *Should one drink only decaffeinated coffee?*

A. Not necessarily. The solvents used to remove caffeine from coffee are often left behind and some of them are known or suspected carcinogens. Studies of decaffeinated coffee indicate that they actually *increase* the output of harmful gastric acids.

Q. *Do you think that caffeine causes fibrocystic disease or breast cancer?*

A. Not at all. I reviewed all of my cases with a proven tissue diagnosis of fibrocystic disease (500 cases) and almost fifty percent drank less than two cups of coffee a day and still got fibrocystic disease. Less than one percent went on to develop breast cancer.

Q. *Are some food additives worse than others?*

A. Definitely. We commonly take in more sodium and sugar than we need and the harmful effects of both are well known. In addition, many of the thousand or more "flavoring agents" in foods are suspected of being cancer-causing substances. These are often complex combinations of ten or more different ingredients.

Q. *What should you look for on a food label?*

A. The amount of fat or protein, sodium and carbohydrates. The Food and Drug Administration requires nutrition information panels only on "enriched" or "fortified" foods or on products that make nutritional claims such as "low-sodium." However, many manufacturers voluntarily list this information even when their products make no special claims.

Q. *What about pesticides and pollutants?*

A. Everyone should be concerned about the environment we live in. The water you drink, the food you eat, the air you breathe; are all precious in their natural state and are necessary to maintain a healthy body. Once they become polluted or chemically changed, they can become harmful and can cause cancer.

11

Stress and the Body's Immune System

If you're one of those people who seldom gets a cold, rarely has the flu and has never had a serious illness, chances are that your body has built up a strong defense system against invading bacteria, viruses and other toxins. More than likely, you pay attention to what you eat, by including plenty of immunity-enhancing foods in your diet. You avoid anxiety, tension and other stressful emotions that are known to drain the immune system. The general ability to fight off disease and infections is governed by the body's immune system and stress is a proven immunity reducer. In research studies so far, it has dramatically lessened the body's disease-fighting powers.

The way the body reacts to stress can vary. Acute stress is known to cause heart attacks and strokes in young and old people. Constant stress can result in peptic ulcers, inflammation of the colon or large bowel (colitis), and changes in the balance of hormones in the body. These reactions are only now becoming understood by physicians and researchers.

Any factor that threatens the health of the body or has an adverse effect on its function can be considered stress—injury, disease, or worry. This concept was first formulated some fifty years ago by Dr. Hans Selye[102] who clarified for countless other scientists the complex relationships between the brain and various endocrine glands and the manner in which they normally function to protect us from both mental and physical stress. The immune system sometimes fails when stress becomes too intense or too prolonged. Numerous studies have been done linking stress to the body's immune system and its cancer-fighting mechanisms. [103,104,105]

THE BODY'S IMMUNE SYSTEM

The immune defenses of your body begin with a "stem cell' in the bone marrow, which produces white blood cells. The white blood cells, called leukocytes, "police" the body in a variety of ways. Some migrate to the thymus gland—a large gland near the heart—where they are programmed by the brain to perform different roles. After leaving the thymus, they are called "T-lymphocytes" and work in two ways: The *helper* cells warn of any intruders or abnormal cells, and the *killer* cells attack the intruder or malignant tissue. Once the intruder is destroyed, the T-lymphocytes stop the process.

Other lymphocytes are programmed outside the thymus and are called B-lymphocytes. They eventually mature into plasma cells, and produce antibodies—chemicals which attack intruding bacteria and viruses. Cancer is believed to evade or somehow alter these defense mechanisms so that uncontrolled division of the abnormal cells occurs and the surrounding tissue is invaded and destroyed. Each individual primary tumor has its own pattern of local behavior and spread—for example, bone metastases are very common in breast cancer but very rare in cancer of the ovary.

The role of stress and its relationship to the immune system is a complicated one. [106,107,108] An extensive network in which specific areas of the brain, in conjunction with the endocrine glands, affect the biological mechanisms that are necessary for host responses is involved. In acute and chronic stress, the adrenal gland releases cortisone which can depress the immune defenses of the body. The degree to which this occurs depends upon the individual—and how that individual copes with the stress.

Other factors affect the immune system as well. [109] Obesity and improper diet greatly lower the cancer-fighting mechanisms, [110,111,112] particularly in breast cancer. In studies of women with breast cancer, a high number were immune-deficient—why they are immune deficient is difficult to determine. Some factors that create immune deficiency states are hormones. Radiotherapy [113] and chemotherapy are known to reduce the T-lymphocytes and suppress the immune system. Prolonged immunosuppressive drugs that are used in organ transplants can suppress the immune system so that a cancer can develop.[114,115] Patients with the AIDS Syndrome eventually become totally immuno-deficient and die from Kaposi's Sarcoma (a cancer).

Not all stress is bad. It can alert the body's defenses so that it can better protect itself against infection, cancer, and other diseases.

There is a small gland at the base of the brain (the pituitary) which plays a key role in the stress syndrome. This gland is the master gland that secretes chemicals (hormones) into the blood stream which affect other glands in the body (adrenal gland, thyroid). The adrenal gland releases cortisone and catecholamines (adrenalin-like substances) (hormones) and these hormones have a pronounced effect on specific organs and tissues. The pituitary-adrenal axis is one of the main reactors when stress from an external stimuli, such as cancer, threatens the human body.

In chronic psychogenic stress, the pituitary-adrenal axis is stimulated excessively and the release of adrenalin-like substances and cortisone has a marked immunosuppressive effect. The blood response B and T-lymphocytes that are necessary for healthy immune responses, are reduced by this chronic psychogenic stress and makes these women more susceptible and vulnerable to get breast cancer.

The pituitary gland also secretes other chemicals that are necessary for a healthy immune system—the growth hormone (GH) and thyroid stimulating hormone (TSH). TSH acts to produce thyroid hormones which is one of the glands necessary to maintain normal healthy metabolic function in the human body. Thyroid disease, particularly hyperthyroidism, is more common in the female and when this occurs the gland frequently hypertrophies (gets bigger) and can easily be seen to be enlarged in the neck. This is felt by some to be a stress response in the gland.

WOMEN AND STRESS

Why are some women more immune than others to breast cancer? Why are they better able to cope with stress? The answer to these related questions can be revealing. Heredity plays a part as does environment and lifestyle. Some women simply can't relax and even when they try the results are unproductive. Few of us really know how to relax or how to benefit from relaxation. The benefits may be considerable indeed, because relaxation can help prevent headaches, hypertension, ulcers, and cancer.

Diet and exercise are important, too. By making wise eating choices, you may be able to fortify your natural defenses and prevent many of the problems that are caused by an immune system breakdown. Studies show exercise is at least as effective as a pill in coping with stress. Women still outnumber men about two to one in taking tranquilizers, but there may be a healthier way of dealing with chronic emotional problems.

Several new studies indicate that exercise releases a chemical substance in the brain called endorphins, which act as a natural tranquilizer. Strenuous exercise—including running, bike riding and jumping rope—relaxes your muscles and makes you less anxious and uptight. Even walking helps. Exercise regularly, at least three times a week, and you may begin to feel more relaxed about yourself and make positive changes in your life, without any harmful side effects. It should also help build up your body to its maximum immunity capabilities.

Even among breast cancer patients, stress has a pronounced effect on immunity and recovery. They worry about whether a lump is benign or cancerous, what kind of surgery they will need, and how it will affect their sexual relationship. The tremendous number of unknowns only adds to existing feelings of anxiety. Among my patients the survival rate was highest (seventy-five percent) among those who exhibited a spirit of willingness and desire to fight the disease and survive. Nearly half of them said they had undergone some stress prior to the diagnosis of breast cancer.

The type of stress was also significant. Family problems or divorce headed the list of stressful situations, followed by alcoholism, loss of loved one, physical or mental illness in family, loss of job, move from home, and depression. Some were not able to handle such stress and it contributed to the onset of breast cancer as the following two case histories illustrate:

A woman with no children, but a supposedly happy marriage, suffers in silence as her husband turns increasingly to alcohol and eventually loses his job. Unable to cope with her chronic stress over his condition, she seeks a divorce and later marries a successful businessman. The business winds up in bankruptcy. She develops cancer of the breast despite having no family history of cancer.

When she is questioned about the lump in her left breast she admits to having noticed it nine months before the mammogram was done, but that her physician told her it was nothing to worry about. A subsequent biopsy revealed an invasive ductal carcinoma with positive hormone receptors. She had a modified mastectomy. This woman has since had breast reconstruction and is alive and well.

In the second case, a young woman with two children suffers through an unhappy marriage, thyroid problems (two operations), a nasty divorce and her mother's death from a stroke at age sixty-one. Following the second operation, she is treated with drugs and told the thyroid gland should be removed eventually. Six years after that is done a lump appears in the left breast and a mammogram reveals a carcinoma. A modified mastectomy with axillary dissection was done and this revealed involvement of the lymph nodes.

There can be no doubt that a lifetime of stress plus the chronic thyroiditis (itself an abnormal immune response) contributed to the onset of breast cancer in this young woman. It is not yet known why the body should lose the ability to distinguish between healthy and malignant tissue, but there is evidence that stress, along with other factors, can be suspected in this destruction of tissues by the body's own antibodies.

TAMING RUNAWAY STRESS

It is impossible to measure the negative influence of stress in our society, but many physicians, including myself, believe that stress, through biological mechanisms, enhances the risk of serious illness ranging from heart attack to cancer. Not everyone can afford long-term psychotherapy to help alleviate stress or anxiety. However, here are proven methods of nonmedical intervention that can be used by anyone to tame runaway stress and its consequences.

Meditation is a proven stress reducer. In every study so far, it has dramatically reduced anxiety in the majority of subjects. Begin by meditating five minutes a day, and increase gradually until you can comfortably meditate for twenty minutes. While meditating, your mind will remain alert, but your heart and respiration rate will drop to what it would be after seven hours of sleep. When you complete your daily meditation, you'll feel more alert, refreshed and able to cope.

Anger can help fight cancer too. In my study of patients with breast cancer, those women who were visibly angry about having cancer—

they openly resented the disease—seemed to survive longer than patients who tried to cope with their cancer by showing a brave face to the world. By releasing their anger, these cancer patients may have also provoked changes in their body chemistry that helped fight the disease.

Wackiness. When periods of stress and symptoms of tension arise, some psychologists believe that it is healthier to stop worrying and to take a completely different tack. We've all got a bit of outrageousness lurking beneath our sometimes overly controlled exteriors, and it can be healthy and tension-relieving to let a little of it surface. Anything will do as long as it's fun but harmless to yourself and others. Breaking out of your normal routine through a little harmless wackiness isn't difficult. Most importantly, it can help you take the world and yourself less seriously and, by doing so, ease some of those stressful feelings.

Hobbies. Brains, like bodies, need exercise if they are to function properly and control stressful situations. Don't be afraid to try something new, completely off your beaten path—like needlepoint, painting, sculpting, or any of a number of hobbies you always wanted to try. Start an indoor garden. Buy an aquarium. Do anything out of the norm you want to—but do it regularly. Many women feel guilty when they're not doing something productive, but the experts reassure us that recreation is not inactivity at all and is not self-indulgent. In fact, it could be an important key to safeguarding your mental and physical health.

Tranquilizers. During the past several years, there has been a growing concern about the indiscriminate use of tranquilizers. While these drugs do not necessarily have a place in the treatment of all patients experiencing stress or who have anxious moments in their life, it is likewise important to recognize that stress is a major health hazard and no woman should be made to feel guilty or inferior by taking them in prescribed doses. Open and trusting communication between you and your doctor regarding the use of these medications, their limitations, and their hazards is essential, however.

SUMMARY/QUESTIONS

Whatever uses will be found for interferon and other stimulants of the body's immune system, will doubtless come, as will every other tool of cancer prevention and treatment, out of a growing number of studies in endocrinology and immunology. Theories, some wildly imaginative, still outnumber facts in many areas. Only when a way has been found to destroy the last cancer cell in the last victim can it truly be said that the science of cancer care is complete. Until that time you can start making adjustments in your diet, exercise and everyday living habits that will build up your body and mind to maximum immunity capabilities.

Q. *Are there any easy ways to combat stress?*

A. Definitely, despite all that has been written about the subject, it remains poorly understood. The bottom line on stress management is to do what makes you feel better. Try taking a hot bath or a fifteen-minute walk. It can do more good to an unhappy but otherwise healthy person than all the medicine and psychology in the world.

Q. *How can one go about avoiding stress?*

A. Not all stress can be avoided, it's an inescapable part of everyday life. However, acute or chronic stress is something to look for and correct. Ask yourself if your expression is always serious, or if you have a frown on your face even when relaxing. Do you often clench your fists or jaw, or frequntly seem worried or preoccupied with one problem or another? Why not express the feelings you have openly and learn to accept them without guilt?

Q. *Does heredity play a role in immunity?*

A. To a degree. Some inherited diseases such as colon polyps and hypogammaglobulinemia are known to impair the body's immune system, although there can also be acquired defects when there is no family history. There is a higher risk of cancer in these patients.

Q. *What is meant by active and passive immunity?*

A. When the individual herself has made the substances that will protect her from disease she is said to have active immunity. When we speak of passive immunity, we mean the immunity developed through injection of "antibodies" which have been created in the body of another person or the laboratory. Passive immunity usually doesn't last very long.

Q. *Can immunotherapy be used to treat breast cancer?*

A. Certainly. No other branch of oncology or cancer treatment has expanded more rapidly nor produced more profound effects upon the control of this disease. Our knowledge about the agents used to stimulate the immune system has had the "side effect" of revealing to scientists and clinicians vast new areas inviting exploration.

Q. Are there many such immunostimulant drugs?

A. Yes, but not all display sufficient anti-tumor activity to prescribe them routinely. The broader hope, obviously, is that some as yet undiscovered chemical agents, synthetic hormones, or immune enhancing agents may prove capable of producing much longer or even permanent remissions, not only of breast cancers but of other forms of cancer as well.

12
Helping Yourself
After Breast Surgery

An individual's personality, rather than age, determines her ability to
recover from the physical and psychological effects of breast surgery.
Many doctors are likely to assume that a woman past menopause will
not miss a breast. A woman in her seventies told me after mastectomy
that she felt like she'd "lost a good friend."

Defense mechanisms, activated or reactivated by surgery, prove in-
adequate for some women. They later regret and resent giving their
consent for the operation. Others report a sense of life "standing still"
or being divided into "before" and "after" phases. They are unable to
concentrate on the future until the crisis abates and they dare to hope
again.

Who are the survivors—those women who remain fully employed
and socially active despite chemotherapy or radical treatment? For the
most part, they are verbal, confrontive, at times scrappy. They can be
hostile, compulsive and demanding upon occasion. Rarely are they
docile or obsequious. The woman who wants to live and wants to fight
will lick the problem. She is unwilling to give up. She will not accept
the alternative.

Among those factors predisposing and perhaps most agreed upon as
personality characteristics of cancer patients who have trouble coping
are: A tendency to hold resentment and marked inability to forgive.

94

Many of these women have a very poor self image and some of them are unable to develop and maintain meaningful long-term relationships. Their grief is usually a prolonged one and they find it difficult to return to the daily chores and resume a normal lifestyle.

Women suffer needlessly as a result of post-operative treatment because their physicians have unknowingly encouraged such negative reactions. When a physician says, in effect, "This may make you sick," many women dutifully follow their doctor's suggestion and proceed to get sick.

It is extremely important for a woman who has a potential serious breast problem to have confidence in the doctor that she has selected to take care of her. There should be a strong bond and the doctor patient relationship should be a healthy one.

It appears that women who do not like their doctors, or who do not really have faith in the efficacy of the treatment they are getting, tend to become sicker than those who are involved in a working partnership with their physicians. They are also those least likely to follow the physician's directions about follow-up care to prevent cancer from recurring.

HOW CANCER CAN SPREAD

In order for a breast cancer patient to better understand how they should examine their body after surgery or other forms of treatment, it is important to know how cancer spreads. For almost a century, breast cancer was thought to be a single disease that progressed in an orderly fashion from the tumor to the lymph nodes in the armpit and, only then, to the rest of the body. Early detection—the discovery of cancer at the earliest possible stage through mammography, breast self-examination, and professional examination—has always been thought to be the best hope of surviving the disease.

Recent research, however, shows that breast cancer may be much more complicated. Some scientists have come to believe that it may well be that breast cancer is a systemic disease from its onset and should be treated as such. Others feel that it starts as a localized disease, a cancer cell that has gone haywire in a localized area and multiplies and grows locally. If treated adequately at that time by surgery, radiation, chemotherapy or a combination of methods, the cancer can be destroyed. The cancer, then does not progress on to involve the lymph glands or spread to other organs.

According to the earlier concept of tumor spread, a radical mastectomy, which always included removal of the axillary lymph nodes, was the logical treatment. The wider surgical excision and the more tissue you removed locally around the breast with the chest wall muscles, a better chance for cure was obtained. The nodes under the armpit were always removed to prevent further metastases (tumor spread). If your operation failed, it was because you were not radical enough.

The care of the breast cancer patient has evolved into multiple choices today because we are detecting breast cancer earlier (minimal cancers) and if that minimal cancer is localized, then the breast can be preserved. The problem is that with our sophisticated methods of detection, we are still unable to determine if the breast cancer is localized and which patient qualifies for breast conservation surgery. This is why there are major controversies about treatment methods and this causes important implications for the effectiveness of post-operative breast cancer care.

The introduction of lumpectomy followed by radiation therapy has introduced a new dimension in follow-up care. It is not easy to follow these patients.

There is no question that any patient who finds a new lump should report it to her physician. The chances are that it may be one of several types of lumps or bumps that are quite natural and benign (Chapter 4). However, it is not unusual for the recovering patient to become panicky and worry about the cancer recurring or spreading with all the attendant fears. She needs to be reassured and, fortunately, there are today a number of tests to do just that. The patient can also be taught what to look for—and told that even if cancer recurs it can be successfully treated.

Often breast cancer patients are not told everything they should know about their condition in the mistaken belief that it will cause them undue anxiety. This jeopardizes follow-up treatment and gives such women a false sense of security. Some don't like the physician who treated them, and may not seek his advice at all. This makes it important for the patient to choose a professional to see after treatment, and one whom she can talk with freely: family doctor, gynecologist, obstetrician, internist, or surgeon.

If her doctor has not already done so, he can refer her to one of the organizations, such as the American Cancer Society's Reach to Recovery Program, that consists of volunteers who have undergone breast surgery. Many of the books written by women and for women that deal with the emotional side effects of breast cancer also can be comforting—and informative. Those who have lost a breast and have related their feelings in books include television correspondent Betty Rollin,[116] former first lady Betty Ford, and actress Ingrid Bergman.

WHAT ARE THE SYMPTOMS?

Most of the patients in my practice seem to want to know more about their disease and what they can do to prevent its recurrence. They are told that tumor spread occurs in three ways: localized invasion of tissue at the site of the operation, through the lymph channels or bloodstream, or across body cavities such as the pleural or peritoneal spaces. Each individual primary tumor has its own pattern of metastasis—for example, bone metastasis is very common in breast cancer.

Once in a while, you run into a problem. Not all patients can emotionally accept the fact that they may get a local recurrence or spread of their breast cancer to other parts of their bodies. This type of patient has to be seen more often to give reassurance and the details of where to look for danger are withheld. The majority of women readily accept that they have a serious problem and can be taught where to look for local recurrences, regional, or distal spread.

A woman who has a small cancer of the breast usually does not have to be seen as often in follow-up as a woman who presents with a large cancer (larger than 4 cm.).

If a woman has a large cancer, she should be seen more frequently since she is at greater risk for local, regional, or systemic spread. What this means is that the doctor following the patient (Oncologist) should be selective in how he follows the breast cancer patient after surgery, since certain types of breast cancer are more serious than others.

LOCAL RECURRENCES

It is difficult to define what is meant by a local tumor recurrence of breast cancer because the controversy develops as to whether one is dealing with a local tumor recurrence or residual disease (disease left behind) or a spread (metastases).

If a mastectomy has been done there are specific areas that a woman should look for local tumor recurrence. The site of the surgery should be inspected routinely on a monthly basis by looking at the wound in the mirror and gently palpating the surface of the chest wall to feel for any small nodules that may be under the skin surface. If a nodule develops the doctor should be notified, since a definitive diagnosis is a simple thing to do by injecting a local anesthetic and removing the nodule for tissue analysis.

Don't panic when this happens. Most of these nodules are benign, and may be small lumps associated with the previous operation (such as silk or other suture material). The lump can be right along the scar and can be a keloid or excessive scar formation.

If a woman has a large advanced cancer of the breast, one can predict a much higher incidence of local tumor recurrence. The size of the lesion, stage of the disease and whether the glands are involved at the initial treatment, all are important.

Sometimes it is difficult to detect local recurrence because of special circumstances. The side-effects of chemotherapy and radiation treatments, can cause the skin to thicken and mask a secondary tumor. Patients who have had such treatment should be seen more frequently by the physician and have mammograms more often.

The woman who has had breast reconstructive surgery, whether soon after mastectomy or later, should also be examined on a regular basis since it is virtually impossible to examine the chest wall and tissue by breast self-examination because of the implant. Most studies[117] of breast cancer patients agree that if the disease recurs at all, it will happen within three years after treatment. However, in my experience tumors have recurred in patients as long as ten years after treatment.

TREATMENT OF LOCAL RECURRENCE

Solitary chest wall tumor recurrences, if small enough, can be treated by surgical excision if the surgeon can cut around the lesion with clear margins. Surgery and radiation therapy has to be used if this can not be accomplished. If there are multiple nodules, systemic drugs (chemotherapy) may have to be added also.

The local recurrent tissue should always be sent for hormone receptor levels no matter what the previous receptor levels show. The receptor levels can change and this could have an influence on treatment methods.

If the lump turns out to be a local recurrence of the cancer, the patient should be worked up to be sure that the lungs, bones, and liver are not involved.

Large local tumor recurrences around the sternum that are resistant to radiation therapy have been surgically resected with some success and salvage.[118]

REGIONAL RECURRENCE OF BREAST CANCER

Regional tumor recurrence of breast cancer implies that the recurrence develops in the drainage area of the breast cancer and that lymph node spread has occurred. The anatomical distribution of sites for lymph node spread has been previously discussed and although most of the lymph drainage goes to the axilla (armpit) drainage also goes to the internal mammary chain of lymph nodes (under the sternum) and can also go to the supraclavicular areas of lymph node spread (above the clavicle).

If a tumor recurrence develops in any of these drainage areas, a lump usually forms and can sometimes be felt by the patient. Women are advised to feel these areas periodically for early detection of trouble.

In order to detect spread to these areas sophisticated x-ray imaging techniques have to be used sometimes since simple palpation or feel by the patient or doctor is not always accurate. Lymphoscintigraphy (x-ray) is not completely accurate either but can be helpful, particularly in imaging the lymph nodes under the sternum (the internal mammary chain).

One should not discourage a patient from examining the drainage areas themselves, however, because good salvage can be obtained with early detection. The patients are advised to check themselves when they are taking a shower, for instance. Many women will be the first to pick up a suspicious lump before their doctor will.

EVALUATION OF LYMPH NODE SPREAD

If a new lump is found in the drainage area of the breast (axilla (armpit) or supraclavicular area) a needle aspiration of the lump can be done to examine the tissue. This can be done by the surgeon in his office under local anesthesia and then the cytopathologist can examine the tissue to determine if a spread has occurred.

Sometimes enlarged glands develop around the root of the lung that will be seen and may be suspicious and the radiologist, under x-ray control, will introduce a long needle to sample the tissue for analysis. This avoids an operation for diagnosis.

TREATMENT OF REGIONAL TUMOR RECURRENCE

If a woman is unfortunate and regional tumor recurrence has developed, the news isn't always that bad and certain further diagnostic steps should be taken. Once lymph node spread of the breast cancer develops, a complete work-up should be done to rule out systemic spread (CAT scans, liver surveys, blood tests, etc.) before treating the patient. The usual treatment for regional spread of breast cancer is chemotherapy or radiotherapy or both and good results can be obtained.

SYSTEMIC SPREAD OF BREAST CANCER

Systemic spread of breast cancer means that bits of the primary cancer have broken off and been carried via the lymph channels or bloodstream to other parts of the body. When this happens the news is not good— fifty percent of patients will not survive unless treatment is begun immediately.[119] The bones are the most common site of systemic spread, followed by the lungs, liver, and brain. Symptoms are both variable and difficult to detect, which is why physicians see such patients on a frequent basis.

Back pain that persists, aching or painful joints, colds or respiratory ailments, and weight loss are signs of systemic illness that patients are advised to check for. Once detected they should not give up hope, however.

Systemic spread of breast cancer is the most serious type, and cure rates are half that of local or regional metastasis. They have also not changed dramatically in the past fifteen years even though we hear constantly about eighty percent of breast cancer patients surviving. The woman that falls into that eighty percent category is usually a woman with a small cancer that was detected early and showed no evidence of tumor spread. Unfortunately, many women when first seen, show evidence of systemic spread and the survival rate drops precipitously (15–25%).

There's reason to believe, however, that these dismal numbers will change in the very near future with advances in chemotherapy and immunotherapy. Monoclonal antibodies, for example, produced in the body, reproduced in test tubes and then injected into the body may be able to seek out and destroy cancer cells. Other anticancer drugs such as interferon and interleukin also show promise as disease fighters with the ability to prevent the spread of cancer.

GETTING THE HELP YOU NEED

Not all therapy for the breast cancer patient is medical. Physical therapists can help mastectomy patients with severe swelling or aching muscles to regain the use of their arms. Mild exercises combined with deep breathing, relaxation and massage can strengthen the arm and extend its range of movement in a short period of time. For women who lack the money or opportunitvy for either breast reconstruction or private therapy, the YWCA has pioneered a low-cost program called Encore, that combines rhythmic exercise, swimming, counseling, and clothing advice for mastectomy patients (Appendix E).

Other support groups help by sharing the experiences and concerns of women who have had breast cancer. Several of them have chapters across the country to help patients and families cope with cancer, improve their quality of life, and combat prejudice against cancer patients. The National Cancer Institute has also funded several projects to study the psychological aspects of breast cancer, including community education, physician education, and crisis counseling. (The psychology of cancer is discussed in more detail in Chapter 14 along with how to cope with the disease.)

Hotlines also exist to answer calls about breast cancer research, diagnosis and treatment. One of them, the Cancer Information Service of the National Cancer Institute (800-422-6237), has trained staff members or volunteers that supply accurate and confidential answers to cancer-related questions, and will often mail free publications that are updated regularly. This hotline is also affiliated with the American Cancer Society and regional cancer centers such as Memorial Sloan-Kettering Cancer Center in New York City.

SUMMARY/QUESTIONS

Until medicine gains a better understanding of the various causes of breast cancer, early detection programs should be acknowledged as providing only limited help. Every woman, and particularly women with breast cancer, need information at one time or another about how breast cancer spreads and treatments to prevent or stop it. The increasing availability of breast-sparing surgery, if they qualify, should encourage women to obtain such information, whether from their family physician, cancer specialist, or support organization. The informed woman usually detects breast cancer early and gets a good result.

Q. How do you define a minimal breast cancer?

A. I define this as a tumor that is 5mm. in size or smaller and usually cannot be felt by palpation (feel) of the breast. Almost all minimal cancers are detected by imaging devices (mammography, xeromammography). These are the women that I feel may qualify for breast conservation surgery (lumpectomy, etc.).

Q. What do you mean by a large breast cancer?

A. Generally, a large breast cancer is a tumor bigger than one and a half inches in diameter. After surgery these patients should be watched more closely since regional or systemic spread of the disease is a greater threat. As a breast cancer increases in size, the risk of spread increases.

Q. How can you tell if the cancer has recurred?

A. By mammography and biopsy to determine if the lump is benign or malignant. Other tests such as bone scans, chest x-rays, CAT scans, ultrasound, nuclear magnetic resonance machines are used as aids in detecting recurrence. It is not easy sometimes to detect early recurrence.

Q. Should I have my ovaries out to prevent cancer recurrence?

A. Probably not. It was once thought that by removing the ovaries, breast cancer would not recur. This did not prove to be true. However, surgery for removal of the ovaries or adrenal glands in those women who had estrogen dependent tumors with recurrence did increase survival time and gave good palliation. Newer estrogen blocking drugs have replaced the need for this type of surgery.

Q. Who should take estrogen-blocking drugs?

A. They are generally prescribed for women with evidence of cancer spread and are also used as a preventative for recurrence. Tamoxifen is the least toxic and is an oral medication that has few side-effects. Tumors that are estrogen-dependent are easier to treat than those that are not. Tamoxifen has been most effective in the post menopausal female.

Q. What other drugs prevent the spread of cancer?

A. Cytoxic agents destroy cancer cells by inhibiting cell division, but dosage must be carefully controlled to protect normal cells, particularly in bone marrow, skin and fetal tissue. Other drugs being investigated include Interferon, 5-Fluorouracil and Melphalan.

Q. *Where can anyone find out about support groups?*

A. Both the American Cancer Society and National Cancer Institute have offices in a number of cities, and you can call their toll-free hotlines for additional information (Appendix E). The YWCA and other local organizations may also offer support and counseling services.

13

Breast Reconstruction After Mastectomy

Artists, for centuries, have considered the female form to be the ultimate in beauty. Their attempts to duplicate it in painting or sculpture are among our most prized possessions. Even these artistic reproductions are not the same as the original object.

Nobody can comprehend the tremendous psychological trauma that occurs when a woman is told she must lose her breast. When this happens, the common feeling is that of being "half a woman" and unattractive to a male partner. One way that women attempt to cope with this real or imagined fear is to seek breast reconstruction. Sometimes the result can turn a woman's life around.

Breast cancer surgeons working with plastic surgeons have recognized the need to help these women who have had a mastectomy. During the past decade numerous new sophisticated plastic procedures have been devised that replace the mound in the breast so that a woman can feel complete again and resume a normal lifestyle.

Unfortunately, not every woman with a mastectomy can qualify for breast reconstruction for both physical and psychological reasons. Almost fifty percent of women with breast cancer when first seen will present with regional glandular spread or spread to other areas of the body and may not qualify. About ten percent of women with breast cancer will present with minimal cancer, that is, cancer with tumors small enough to be eligible for possible limited surgery (lumpectomy or quadrectomy).

The good news is that with the new imaging techniques (mammography, xeromammography, etc.) more and more small tumors are being detected and fewer mastectomies may need to be done in the future.

Approximately seventy percent of women with breast cancer that does not show spread, still require some form of mastectomy, not all of which leave the woman physically capable of having her breast restored. There is also the question of whether reconstructive surgery can produce the sought after psychological effects the patient seeks.

This is a matter of no small concern among cancer specialists and plastic surgeons who must treat the breast cancer patient in body and spirit. They must attempt to answer her questions and determine the reasons behind them. How will it look? Will the scars go away? What about the nipple? What if the cancer comes back? The woman who desires breast reconstruction has to face all of these considerations squarely.

HOW PATIENTS ARE SELECTED

Breast reconstruction isn't anything new. What is new is that there's an easier method now to replace the breast mound—the silicone implant. Surgeons are doing less disfiguring radical mastectomies—so that plastic surgery is possible in more cases. However, such surgery, indeed any further hospitalization, is not for every woman who may have already endured the trauma of cancer, mastectomy, and perhaps radiation therapy.

In my opinion, breast reconstruction remains for the highly motivated woman. Since some health insurance plans unfortunately define any plastic surgery as "elective" or "cosmetic" a woman may need to pay the entire hospital and surgical cost herself. Age need not preclude such an operation, however. Too often the attitude has been, "Why do you want reconstruction? You should be happy just to be alive." My own experience is any woman who wishes reconstruction, and who is suitable for it, should have it.

It has been stated that a woman's physiological age is more important than her chronological age. One should add to that, a woman's psychological age or how a woman can create her own lifestyle. How does a person dress and look? How active is she in daily living? You can be over seventy, but feel and behave like fifty or younger because you are in good physical shape and mental spirits. My oldest "reconstructed" patient was sixty-five years old and the youngest twenty-eight.

Physicians are finally coming to see what many women have been saying all along: Reconstruction can add to a woman's positive feelings about herself. Some women can learn to live without a breast, others cannot. Some will not let their husbands touch them, or see them undressed. They should have the option of reconstruction without having to make excuses for their choice. Some experts on aging even suggest that, if a surgeon turns you down for restorative surgery just because of your age, you should get a second opinion and if necessary a third.

Medically speaking, the selection of patients for breast reconstruction is more clearcut. They should have no evidence of diffuse tumor spread and they should wait a year or more for the mastectomy to heal properly. This also allows for better follow-up examination, since a silicone implant or muscle transposition can make it difficult to detect local recurrence on the chest wall. Most local recurrences occur within the first three years following surgery.[117]

WHICH KIND OF RECONSTRUCTION SHOULD BE DONE?

There are several different procedures that can be done, depending upon the patient's condition and the skill of the surgeon. To help ensure the best results, it is wise to seek a surgeon who is board certified by the American College of Plastic Surgery and who is doing frequent reconstructive breast surgery. You may have to ask around to find out who is doing the best reconstructive surgery in your area. Sometimes, you may have to seek treatment outside your local area.

During the past fifteen years, methods have been devised to recreate the missing mound of the breast with a silicone implant[120,121] or to transfer tissue from a part of the body to another. Skin and muscle flaps with its attached blood supply (myocutaneous flaps) have been used to replace the defect created by mastectomy.[122,123,124] Skin expander techniques and plastic prosthetic devices have been improved.[125,126]

Basically, the idea is to form a pocket into which the silicone gel implant is placed. (See Figure 7) If too much skin or muscle was removed in the mastectomy, a muscle skin flap might have to be created. For the woman with a good base of skin and muscle over the chest wall, implantation and reconstruction is a one-stage procedure. Some

Figure 7

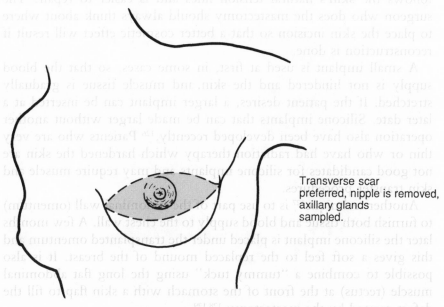

Transverse scar preferred, nipple is removed, axillary glands sampled.

POST MASTECTOMY SILICONE IMPLANT

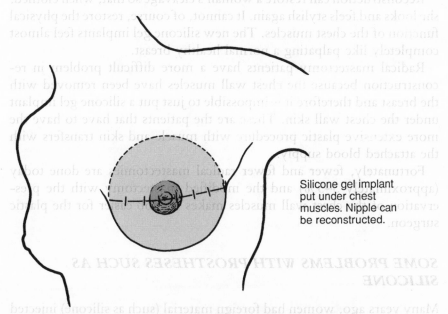

Silicone gel implant put under chest muscles. Nipple can be reconstructed.

SIMPLEST AND MOST POPULAR RECONSTRUCTION
FOLLOWING MASTECTOMY

surgeons are now doing mastectomy with a horizontal incision that follows the skin's natural tension lines and is easier to repair. The surgeon who does the mastectomy should always think about where to place the skin incision so that a better cosmetic effect will result if reconstruction is done.

A small implant is used at first, in some cases, so that the blood supply is not hindered and the skin and muscle tissue is gradually stretched. If the patient desires, a larger implant can be inserted at a later date. Silicone implants that can be made larger without another operation also have been developed recently.[126] Patients who are very thin or who have had radiation therapy which hardened the skin are not good candidates for silicone implants and may require muscle and skin transfer procedures.

Another technique[127] is to use part of the abdominal wall (omentum) to furnish both tissue and blood supply to the chest wall. A few months later the silicone implant is placed under the transplanted omentum and this gives a soft feel to the replaced mound of the breast. It is also possible to combine a "tummy tuck" using the long flat abdominal muscle (rectus) at the front of the stomach with a skin flap to fill the defect created by the mastectomy.[128,129]

Reconstruction can restore a woman's cleavage so that, when clothed, she looks and feels stylish again. It cannot, of course, restore the physical function of the chest muscles. The new silicone gel implants feel almost completely like palpating a normal healthy breast.

Radical mastectomy patients have a more difficult problem in reconstruction because the chest wall muscles have been removed with the breast and therefore it is impossible to just put a silicone gel implant under the chest wall skin. These are the patients that have to have the more extensive plastic procedure with muscle and skin transfers with the attached blood supply.

Fortunately, fewer and fewer radical mastectomies are done today (approximately 3–5%) and the modified mastectomy with the preservation of the chest wall muscles makes the job easier for the plastic surgeon.

SOME PROBLEMS WITH PROSTHESES SUCH AS SILICONE

Many years ago, women had foreign material (such as silicone) injected with a needle into their breasts to increase their breast size or to make them appear firmer. Some of these women went on to develop cancer of the breast. There is no evidence that the silicone implants used in breast reconstruction today cause cancer. The silicone material is placed within a plastic shell. Some of the new silicone gel prostheses have a button into which more material can be injected or removed if the woman wishes a larger or smaller size breast.

Occasionally, a contracture or tightening of the tissue around the implant develops and the new mound is not symmetrical with the other breast. This usually has to be taken care of surgically.

There is also the possibility of silicone leaking from the prosthesis. I saw a woman who developed a lump next to her silicone prosthesis and she was extremely apprehensive about possible recurrent cancer. A mammogram was done and the radiologist, who examined her, felt that the lump was silicone that had leaked from her prosthesis and this was confirmed when the implant was removed and another inserted.

There has been some controversy concerning breast reconstruction, and this is advice for any woman considering it:

1) Ask to talk with and see other women who have had breast reconstruction. Remember results are not always the same for different women with different tumors.
2) Understand that there are several types of operations and implants. Ask the surgeon to discuss the advantages and disadvantages of each.
3) Ask the surgeon how many reconstructions he or she has done.
4) Ask to see pictures. Some surgeons do not give out names of patients, but you should be able to look at "before" and "after" photographs of women who have had reconstruction.

SUMMARY/QUESTIONS

If you want reconstruction, the time to speak up is before a mastectomy. In the past so many women got hostile reactions from their physicians that they became discouraged. This has changed today and reconstructed breasts can be quite natural-looking. The woman with an implant or muscle skin graft should know, however, that follow-up examination is both necessary and can be more difficult.

Q. What is your criteria for selection of patients for reconstruction?

A. The method of selection of patients for reconstruction should have a strict criteria and the patients should be completely free of metastatic disease. The limits and risks should be discussed openly with the patient. Reconstruction should not be offered to all mastectomy patients and not all mastectomy patients are interested in having it done.

I advise them to wait for about a year before the reconstruction. This allows the skin flap to heal properly and allows the blood supply to grow into the area. It also allows for shoulder motion to return to normal. Most patients that request reconstruction of the breast are the younger sexually active patients and not the older postmenopausal patients. Age should not be a barrier, however, for reconstruction of the breast if the patient is in good health.

Q. What about patients with regional spread who want reconstruction?

A. I prefer that reconstruction of the breast be done on those patients with minimal cancer that show no evidence of regional or systemic spread. An exception to that is a patient with regional spread who has survived for over three years without evidence of progression of their disease.

Q. In some sections of the country immediate reconstruction of the breast is offered to the patient prior to mastectomy. How do you feel about that?

A. I usually do not advocate immediate reconstruction of the breast. The most important reason is that the breast cancer surgeon should be concentrating on doing a good cancer operation and should not be thinking about how he should be reconstructing the breast. It is important that the breast cancer tissue and the axillary nodes be analyzed before a decision is made about reconstruction. If many of the glands are positive, I do not advise the procedure.

Q. Can complications occur after immediate reconstruction?

A. Yes, sometimes a wound infection or slough of tissue may develop causing the loss of the skin covering of the breast and a major complication can be overwhelming since postoperative bleeding can also develop. I prefer that the patient adjust to the loss of the breast and have delayed reconstruction of the breast if they have a reasonable life expectancy.

Q. Are there any other considerations concerning immediate reconstruction?

A. Some women today are given adjuvant chemotherapy or radiation therapy or both as part of the regimen of their treatment. This should be completed prior to reconstruction.

Q. *Which women with breast cancer do you advise not to have reconstruction?*

A. Those patients in which numerous lymph glands are found to be involved with metastatic cancer. Patients with diffuse metastatic cancer of the breast to the bones, brain, and lungs are also discouraged from having reconstruction. Those women with serious medical problems are also advised against it.

Q. *How should you work up a patient prior to reconstruction?*

A. It should be determined that no evidence of local or metastatic disease is present before embarking on reconstruction. A chest x-ray, bone scan, liver scan, and if necessary, a CAT scan of the brain should be done to rule out spread. One cannot be definitely sure, even with modern testing, that systemic breast cancer is not present.

Q. *How do you select a plastic surgeon for your mastectomy patients?*

A. I usually give the patient the names of three plastic surgeons so that they may select their own. I prefer a plastic surgeon who is willing and capable of doing all types of procedures and avoid those that limit themselves to one or two procedures. I also prefer those who are doing breast surgery frequently in order to get good cosmetic results.

Q. *What are the advantages and disadvantages of the various reconstructive methods after mastectomy?*

A. All of our cancer patients were asked how they felt about the breast reconstruction that they had done. We also asked them whether they would have the procedure done again. The patients that were pleased with their reconstruction were the patients that had the simplest procedures such as the silicone implant. The answer that they gave was that they no longer had to worry about that "thing" (external breast prosthesis) being placed in the right place. They felt that their body contour was more normal.

Q. *What did the patients with breast reconstruction object to the most?*

A. The main objection to reconstruction came from patients who had musculocutaneous (muscle-skin) island flaps. The latissimus dorsi myocutaneous flap was objected to the most. This is the muscle on the flank and back that is used. Many said they would not have it done again. They did not like the scar on the back and the restriction of movement associated with the flap. They objected to the two or three procedures needed for the reconstrucion and to the operation (reduction mammoplasty) that often had to be done on the remaining breast. Some patients objected to the economic cost and others to the multiple scars created by the muscle transposition.

Q. *Should the nipple be removed when doing a mastectomy?*

A. One of the major objections to doing a mastectomy and removing the nipple is that in reconstruction of the breast the woman wishes that a new nipple be made. The new nipple is never as good as the original. Most breast cancers are infiltrating ductal cancers and the ducts connect with the nipple. If the nipple is left behind the patient is at risk to getting local recurrence at the site of the retained nipple. This means that a rigid criteria has to be used in selecting patients who may qualify for the preservation or banking of the nipple at another site and then using it later in the reconstrucion.[130,131]

Q. *Should the reconstructed breast be symmetrical with the remaining breast?*

A. Sometimes this is difficult to achieve because the patient may have a large remaining breast and a reduction in size (reduction mammoplasty) of the remaining breast has to be done. Since the second breast is at increased risk to getting cancer, an argument can be made for removing the breast tissue in that breast followed by a silicone implant.

Q. *Are there any complications to breast reconstruction after mastectomy?*

A. Yes, but as more and more of these procedures are done experience is gained and less complications occur. In the cases that I have seen most of the complications have occurred in the irradiated cases and in those patients who have had the radical mastectomy with removal of the muscles prior to reconstruction. In the zeal to attempt to eradicate the cancer by surgical means, little soft tissue and thin skin remains for an adequate reconstruction. Pre-operative irradiation (prior to reconstruction) reduces the normal circulation to the area and one is more apt to get a slough of the skin flap. Patients with hematological disorders or blood clotting deficiencies are also more apt to get a hematoma (collection of blood) which may lead to an infection and a resultant loss of the implant.

Q. *Can radiation therapy be given after a silicone implant?*

A. Yes, and I find that radiation therapy is being used more and more as an adjunctive method of treatment with surgery, particularly when a minimal cancer is found. Chemotherapy is being used more often for those premenopausal breast cancer patients that have more than three lymph glands positive.

Q. *Please elaborate more on local recurrence and breast reconstruction.*

A. It is not easy to follow a patient who has had a reconstruction of the breast after mastectomy. If there is a silicone bag or prosthesis between the chest wall and the surface skin it is almost impossible to determine if a recurrence has developed beneath the prosthesis. This also applies if a patient has had a musculocutaneous flap or island flap that covers up the defect created by removing the breast.

Local recurrence is an extremely important fact to consider whenever one considers breast reconstruction. The number of cases that recur is related to the size and type of tumor. If the tumor is small and low-grade, the chance of recurrent disease decreases. If the tumor is large and aggressive, or if there are many lymph glands involved in the axilla (armpit) the chance of local recurrence increases and can be as high as 30–45%. Most studies done on local recurrence have been done on patients following radical mastectomy.

The usual local recurrence rate is about 10–20%. That rate increases based on the length of time the patient is followed. I have had patients develop local recurrence at six years, eleven years, and fourteen years.

Q. *Some doctors have recommended removal of breast tissue (subcutaneous mastectomy) to prevent cancer. Others have advocated mastectomy as a preventative measure in specific types of precancerous lesions. How do you feel about that?*

A. The subject of attempting to remove all breast tissue to prevent cancer of the breast has been discussed and written about for many years.[132] The basic problem that has to be faced, however, is whether 100% of the breast tissue can be removed when doing a prophylactic subcutaneous mastectomy because if tissue is left behind that tissue is at risk to get cancer and may be at an increased risk.

Q. *Can you remove all the breast tissue when you do a subcutaneous mastectomy?*

A. This is the crux of the problem. It is impossible to remove all of the breast tissue; breast tissue is always left behind under the nipple and in the tail of spence (axillary tail). Small pieces of breast tissue are scattered under the skin flaps also. The breast is a secreting organ (lactation, milk) and if breast tissue is left behind that tissue is still going to be affected by hormones (estrogen, progesterone) and can cause problems.

Q. *Should a woman discuss costs before having reconstructive procedures done on the breast?*

A. Yes, I tell the patient to discuss costs with the plastic surgeon and to ask about the various options of treatment and the number of procedures needed to accomplish the desired result. In some states the cost of reconstruction of the breast after mastectomy is paid for by health insurance, but not in all states. The cost of reconstruction can be quite expensive in some areas.

Q. *How much does breast reconstruction cost?*

A. Anywhere from $3,000 to $10,000 depending upon the number of procedures that have to be done and where it is done. You should check with your physician and your insurance company about whether your surgery qualifies for insurance coverage before you have your reconstruction done.

Q. *Where can one get advice and counseling before breast reconstruction?*

A. The Reach to Recovery Program of the American Cancer Society can provide information to women interested in breast reconstruction after mastectomy. Volunteers who have had reconstruction are available to visit women who are deciding about this type of surgery. No products are endorsed and there is no charge for this service. Some breast surgeons have their own mastectomy patients, who have had successful reconstructions, that work with the doctor in counseling women who may request reconstruction.

Q. *Which patients are most unhappy with reconstruction?*

A. Those who have a poor self-image to begin with, and expect the surgery to change their life. They also may have emotional problems unrelated to the physical disease that can only be resolved through counseling or psychotherapy.

14
Quality of Survival—
Coping with Breast Cancer

Not many years ago, if a woman went into the hospital for a breast tumor biopsy the surgeon would remove the suspicious lump and a frozen section analysis of the tissue would be done. If the pathologist said a cancer was present the surgeon would usually procede with a radical mastectomy. The patient actually had very little choice or option in her treatment.

Fortunately, today, a two-step procedure is done. The biopsy is done first. A diagnosis is made and then the woman participates in discussion of the numerous options of care. The breast cancer specialist tries to fully inform her about alternative methods of treatment.

Informed consent means exactly what it says. It means that the patient wishes to be fully informed or instructed comprehensively about her options in treatment in order to select the method that she wants to be used on her. After being fully informed, if that is possible, she then consents to the treatment. (See Chapter 7)

Major operations are a traumatic experience for the individual going under the knife and a mastectomy is no exception. An important sexual organ is being removed and the woman's body is altered and a new body image must be rebuilt.

The immediate adaptation to this experience will vary with each individual. The older female seems to adapt better to the loss of her breast than the younger one. It is harder for a young female to accept the insult that a mastectomy has on her body. Usually she is sexually active and she worries about her sexual relationship with her partner. There are many myths abut the mastectomy patient and the most common is the feeling of being half a woman and no longer being sexually attractive to the male partner.

There is no doubt that there is a body contour change when the breast is removed, but how that affects the love relationship should be debated. I asked all of my mastectomy patients if their sexual relationship had changed after mastectomy. Twenty percent said that it had changed for the worse. Some of these women blamed themselves. They said it was not due to the male partner's ardor but rather due to their own emotional readjustment. They said they became depressed, withdrawn, and unable to continue their daily chores adequately. They were lacking in self esteem and often refused the supportive gestures of family and friends.

Actually, if the man and woman have a strong relationship prior to mastectomy, that relationship continues and many times the male becomes more considerate and affectionate.

I find that the quicker the woman faces the reality of the mastectomy, the quicker the adjustment is made. To ignore the situation—to treat the woman as though nothing has happened, can be psychologically damaging. She cannot then unburden herself of her feelings and this repression may delay recovery.

Love and communication are the basic ingredients in a good family relationship, and when these are present, the shape or absence of breasts becomes unimportant. The brush with death itself often brings couples closer together.

Many husbands and lovers, after initial shock, respond to their partners nobly. A tall, pretty stockbrocker that I did a mastectomy on when she was twenty-nine years old, was depressed following her surgery because she felt she would never have the chance to marry after having the mastectomy. Fortunately, she got married at the age of thirty-two and now has two lovely children of her own. She told me that her sexual relationship is completely normal and happy.

Another woman, sixty, told me that she missed her breast and was considering reconstruction, "Women live a lot longer than men you know . . . If my husband dies it will help make me more attractive and appealing." Others do not respond or adjust this well.

This is especially true for the unmarried or divorced, who expect that the loss of a breast will cost them dearly. Sometimes it does, but not in the numbers one would suppose. Consider, for example, the following case history of an attractive young woman, forty-one, whose lover "took off as soon as my mastectomy was done."

She was separated from her husband at the time of the operation and had expressed some doubts about how her new partner would react, since he had told her on more than one occasion that her breasts were beautiful. When asked how she felt now, she said, "It was the best thing that ever happened to me. One boob is not something on which to base a marriage. Incidentally, my husband is in the waiting room. Would you like to meet him?"

One patient's husband told me, after his wife's mastectomy, that when he looked at his wife, he didn't think of her as missing a breast but missing the cancer or tumor that had been in her body. The fact that she had only one breast didn't make him love her any less. He was grateful for the fact that the cancer had been removed from his wife's body.

COPING WITH DEPRESSION

The amount of help a woman gets from her husband, lover or friends usually depends on the prior quality of the relationship. The help she gets is extremely important and usually determines whether she has a short or long depression. Shrouding the operation in secrecy, omitting family members from medical discussions—ignoring a woman's emotions or overprotecting her—any of these stances impedes help. Some women vent their anger on the surgeon who did this to them, and others express denial or disbelief. Often they will need outside counseling if they are to overcome feelings of depression or anxiety. This is not without danger in unqualified hands.

One woman who went to group therapy sessions after her mastectomy came to see me deeply disturbed. She said that a breast patient at one of the sessions told her that she had the "wrong" operation and that she should have had a lumpectomy like she had done. It took some time to convince this patient that she did, indeed, have the right operation for her circumstances, and that only one in ten women qualify for a lumpectomy. The point was really brought home to this patient however, when the woman with the lumpectomy developed a local recurrence and had to have a subsequent mastectomy.

What are some of the ways a woman can help herself cope after a mastectomy? I find that the women who exercise and try to keep their bodies in good shape seem to cope better with the physical and psychological trauma associated with mastectomy. As part of a rest and relaxation treatment, particularly if you're the aggressive, self-driven type, try deep-breathing exercises, walking or biking. They're good for health, for morale—and you won't overdo it.

Regular, self-induced relaxation can also be helpful in beating the blues. One way to help yourself is to try meditation or visualization. These are nothing new. What is new is that many physicians, after focusing for a long time on the body alone, are beginning to pay more attention to the ways in which health is influenced by mental and emotional states. Meditation also helps insomnia. In fact, persons who have difficulty falling asleep, tossing or turning for hours, can usually do so in fifteen minutes when they practice meditation. If you need help, meditation tapes and casettes are available. Ask your doctor about them.

Visualization is a technique first begun by a radiation oncologist[133] to help patients help themselves by changing one's lifestyle either to eliminate stressful situations or cut back on them. It's not mind over matter, or "wishing" one's body to be well. Rather, visualization is maintaining a positive attitude and refusing to allow negative feelings to interfere with one's return to health. Breast cancer is not the only disease for which emotional or stress-related factors are suspected, so it is important for every woman to know and understand this and act accordingly.

PROSTHESIS OR RECONSTRUCTION

No one claims that a few ounces of foam rubber can ever replace a breast, or help somebody live with the fact that she has had cancer. For many women prostheses or external breast forms are a sensible, accepted alternative to further surgery. They can make most women look normal in even the most revealing fashions and feel physically and emotionally complete. Most large department stores and a number of specialty shops carry many wardrobe items for the mastectomy patient, and some are run by women who have had the operation themselves.

Many health insurance plans will pay for breast prostheses, and some women use inexpensive, homemade breast forms. One patient of mine told me that she had tried several prostheses, but found that the one she made herself worked best and looked the most natural. Others found that by wearing loose-fitting but stylish clothing they could present a perfectly normal appearance. What's important is that individuals who are able to adjust their attitudes as well as their lifestyles respond well to recovery and have fewer emotional problems.

My advice to any woman who has had a mastectomy is not to isolate yourself from other people. If you have a hobby, check to see if your local college or night school offers courses in the subject. Investigate social groups that are organized by churches, temples or other private organizations. Make a real effort to broaden your social contacts. If you always eat at home or watch TV alone, try going out to a movie or eating at a restaurant with friends occasionally.

Invariably the woman who has had a breast removed will at least consider reconstruction, particularly those women who are unmarried or divorced. There are several types of operations using implants or other methods that can be done (Chapter 13), but they are all expensive and not without risks. For the woman who is highly motivated, breast reconstruction can be a blessing.

There is no reason to run away from the idea of cancer or avoid treatment. In many instances it can be completely cured, and the lives of some famous women attest to this fact: Julia Child, Shirley Temple Black, Betty Rollin, and, of course, Betty Ford and Happy Rockefeller. All of them continue to be active and productive many years after diagnosis and treatment. Other women have similar stories.

THE QUALITY OF SURVIVAL[134]

"For what is a man profited, if he shall gain the whole world, and lose his own soul?" MATTHEW 16, VERSE 26.

This statement can be applied to the breast cancer patient: "What do we gain if we save a larger number, only to have them lead a life which, for them, is living hell."[134]

If a patient has a breast lump, has a biopsy, and is told she has cancer and may need a mastectomy, what is her quality of life like after her treatment? If we talk about the quality of survival of the breast cancer patient, we have to talk about all the patients afflicted with this disease.

Quality of survival is a determination of how a patient lives and survives after they develop a disease and are treated. The concept has to be debated openly in today's society. If a patient is just alive and does not function or return to work or resume normal body functions and social communication with the family, friends, and the outside world, then the patient does not have a good quality of survival.

There are moral, ethical, and economic questions that have to be answered. The issue not only pertains to the cancer patient, but to all patients with a serious disease.

As to whether the individual affected with breast cancer does have a quality of survival that civilization can be proud of, depends not only on the individual herself, but the doctor treating her, the response of her family to her emotional needs and to the communication and warmth used in working out the trauma associated with breast cancer.

There are many questions that must be answered in regards to the breast cancer patient's quality of life and quality of survival. How does one define quality of survival since each survivor is a different individual and each one may have different values and goals in life?

How does the patient feel about her treatment? Is she healthy? The stage of her disease is important when answering this question since the surgery, radiation, or chemotherapy treatment or combinations of treatment are usually more aggressive the more serious the breast cancer problem.

If the patient is unfortunate and the disease has spread to her regional nodes (lymph glands) or there is systemic spread (bones, lungs, liver, brain, etc.) chemotherapy is often recommended for treatment.

If she needs chemotherapy will she accept this optimistically or will she be depressed and be limited in her ability to get around and return to work or conduct her usual activities as a housewife?

Studies have been done comparing endocrine (hormonal) and cyto-toxic (chemo) therapy in women with advanced breast cancer. If the patients saw that their tumors were responding to treatment, they were able to tolerate the toxic side effects of the chemotherapy, however, if there was no response, the treatment toxicity became unbearable.[135,136] Not all patients will continue with the chemotherapy protocols (treatment). Some patients cannot tolerate the nausea, vomiting or loss of hair that often occurs.

With improved treatments providing better cure rates for breast cancer and increased length of survival, how well do patients do in terms of quality of life after mastectomy or other treatment?

My own research confirms the fact that too much emphasis has been given to cancer as an enigma, and that the quality of survival depends to a great degree upon what has been called the "hopelessness potential"—a psychological scale to measure how much control the women felt they had over their lives, futures and the state of their health. A disproportionate number of breast cancer patients seem to live their lives in an emotional crouch—often feeling helpless, worried and pessimistic. They tend to repress their anger but accept their depressions. They ignore their achievements but embrace their failures.

For a long time, however, these observations were *just* observations—informal suspicions that a person's mental state might somehow play a role in the treatment of cancer. It wasn't until the latter half of this century that these hunches began to harden into scientific theory. The doctors at several university hospitals evaluated women who had to undergo biopsies for breast lumps for signs of depression and other emotional disorders. The results were sobering.

For the women who had been diagnosed as depressed originally, the death rate from cancer was twice as high as the rate found in the general population. Other risk factors—such as obesity or stress—were taken into account in these investigations. However, the depression alone, it was concluded, was a critical factor in the patient's length of survival. The doctors were not looking for depression, but for traumatic life events that may have preceded the development of the disease or followed treatment.

Why should what goes on in our minds be expressed in our cells? The answer may lie in the immune system. In even the healthiest person, scattered cancer cells may occasionally appear and begin to multiply. When the immune system is functioning as it should, white blood cells are able to exterminate the rogue malignancies. If, however, the immune system falters—responds too late or too listlessly—then cancer may have a chance to take hold.

Skeptics question the reliability of these findings. Even doctors who support this type of research admit that diagnosing emotional conditions and establishing their relation to physical health is an imprecise science at best. Does depression really *precede* cancer, or does cancer—even before it's discovered—wrack the body so that subjects begin to feel defeated and depressed without knowing why? Do those who interview women in a hospital environment after a biopsy for breast cancer get a true picture of the subject's feelings of hopelessness or hopefulness?

My own feeling is that a chronically repressed or depressed temperament is a cancer signpost, not a cancer sentence. Most women today *know* that mastectomy is the usual treatment for breast cancer and that the disease is definitely curable. The problem then is whether they believe it—and act accordingly. There are, indeed, reasons for regarding cancer as a serious enemy. They are not reasons for anxiety or depression. Quite the contrary—the killer has not been isolated and destroyed, but it is being cornered. Our knowledge provides us with the weapons to win countless victories, if everyone uses this knowledge.

No longer should any woman feel that she must lose a breast to cancer. If that should become necessary, she should know that her life afterward can be a long and happy one. There is no reason to believe that she can't have children—or that she won't be around to raise the ones she does have.

Those patients who resumed their household duties or returned to work without taking the time to turn inward or contemplate their wound also showed the least depression or hopelessness. Their willingness to fight, in my opinion, had a beneficial effect on the immune system that equaled the power of antitoxic drugs or chemotherapy. They never felt abandoned and even when there was a recurrence that ability to face adversity was crucial to their continued survival.

SUMMARY/QUESTIONS

Cancer patients are hardly benefited by studies that suggest—even obliquely—that they somehow have brought their illness upon themselves. They should know, however, that their emotions can play an important part in early detection, treatment and recovery from the disease. Those that do, have been shown to have high cure rates and successful rehabilitation. Nowhere is psychology as important as in the treatment of cancer with all of its unreasoning fears—and women can, with a little assistance, learn to help themselves fight and conquer these fears.

Q. *Should the patient be told all the details of their cancer or spread of their cancer? Should they be told the truth?*

A. I think you have to listen to the patient. They often will tell you how much or how little and how often they want to talk about their diagnosis and future. The doctor's answers to the patient's questions should be done candidly and should not be embellished. I feel the patient should be told the truth. Most of the time this helps to maintain a good healthy doctor/patient relationship. If the patient, at some point, finds out that the doctor kept some of the facts regarding her diagnosis from her, she may not trust the doctor in the future and it's very important that she have faith in her physician.

Q. *What do you tell women who must undergo a mastectomy?*

A. First off, that saving her life is more important than saving her breast. Then it is possible to discuss the type of surgery, how it may affect breast reconstruction, and results with similar patients. It helps, if the woman is married, to have the husband present at this time so that rehabilitation can begin before surgery.

Q. *What do you tell a woman who has a lumpectomy, axillary dissection and radiation treatment?*

A. I tell them that they are fortunate that they have a minimal cancer and have the option of breast conservation surgery. I also tell them that it will be more difficult to follow them after radiation therapy for local recurrence and that there may be delayed problems from the radiation.

Q. *What do you tell a woman who had a mastectomy followed by breast reconstruction?*

A. These women are also told that it will be more difficult to watch the mastectomy site since a silicone gel prosthesis will be placed over the chest wall.

Q. *Is it natural to be depressed after a mastectomy?*

A. Of course—what isn't natural is to be depressed months later, or to isolate one's self from normal social contact because of the operation. Those patients who adjust best usually do so immediately or within a short period of time. Both doctor and family can be supportive to make this transition easier.

Q. *How can a husband help the mastectomy patient?*

A. By being loving and understanding in his reaction to the operation, and constant in his actions. Many husbands are fearful of doing or saying the wrong thing and this can appear to be rejection when it's not. He can also look for and respond to any clues his partner gives to how she feels.

Q. *Do you prescribe tranquilizers or other drugs?*

A. It depends—certainly, there's no reason not to if the patient has taken such medications in the past, or is actually anxious or in pain. Each case has to be treated individually and, in some instances, psychological counseling may be recommended.

Q. *Why is there such a preoccupation with breasts in our society?*

A. The way we dress; perhaps if women were to wear saris as they do in India or the slit skirts as in the Far East there would not be so much emphasis on a woman's breasts. Women themselves are not blameless in this preoccupation and act according to what fashion demands.

Q. *What can you tell the children?*

A. Not much, if they are quite young. Just the word cancer scares most children, as it does adults, and they may not be old enough to cope with the knowledge. Older children can and should be told about the operation and what it means. In my experience they are often most supportive.

Q. *Why do you emphasize the psychology of cancer?*

A. We have gone about as far as we can in surgical treatment and tend to ignore the rehabilitation of breast cancer patients. As we have seen, the emotions can play an important role in the recovery process and even help prevent recurrence. This, and current experiments with anticancer drugs, are perhaps the most exciting areas of research.

Q. *What do you mean by quality of survival?*

A. How the patient adjusts to her treatment and how it affects her future lifestyle. It is not possible to predict how an individual will respond, but we can offer practical advice and guidance based on the experiences of other women who have had breast cancer.

Q. *Can anything be done for the woman wih advanced breast cancer?*

A. There are a number of promising anticancer drugs that work on the cancer cell and the immune system to prevent the spread of cancer, and scientists are working to lessen their side-effects and make these treatments more bearable.

Q. *What do you tell the woman with advanced cancer who has no chance of survival?*

A. Despite moral, ethical and economic questions, my own feeling is that every patient should have the right to seek and obtain treatment even if it is only palliative. She should not be abandoned to hopelessness and she should be assured that attempts will be made to help her and also to relieve her pain.

Q. *Why do you feel that way?*

A. We are transplanting organs and making artificial ones every day for patients who would otherwise die. New drugs are also being found for diseases once thought incurable, so there is no reason why one or more shouldn't be found for cancer of the breast. Hope and not despair should guide the choice of each patient with cancer.

Q. *How do you feel about cancer insurance?*

A. It can be a good idea for the high-risk patient—and some two million policies are sold each year. The reason is that, per patient, the total medical cost for treating some breast cancers can cost as much as $100,000. Whether cancer insurance provides adequate financial protection is open to question. Some policies pay only a third of hospital costs. Others will not cover complications, or impose a time limit after a cancer is first diagnosed. An alternative might be an "excess major medical" rider to an existing health insurance policy such as catastrophic insurance.

15

The Outlook for the Future

Much of what we know about breast cancer has seemed "forever" but as you have seen in this book, even the entrenched radical mastectomy is giving way to many new breast care options in treatment that can save women's bodies and lives and, in some selected cases, preserve the breast. Researchers in many fields, not just oncology, have contributed to enormous progress in earlier detection (mammography, ultrasound, nuclear magnetic resonance) and as breast cancer is detected when it is small, the treatment can be less radical.

If basic scientists determine that breast cancer is a systemic disease from the onset, new methods of controlling the disease will be developed in the future. Ten years ago, this view would have been ridiculed and few dared to challenge the prevailing wisdom. Controversy sometimes is the only method that stimulates progress.

Now thousands of women are learning about the choices available to them and that breast cancer need not be the dreadful, multilating killer it has been feared to be. Cancer management today is becoming increasingly individualized, both with respect to diagnostic procedures and treatment. Early detection is followed by a precise staging of the disease and the use of more than one kind of therapy, often in combination.

With medical progress producing better cure rates and longer survival

126

periods, concerns are expanding to include the woman's psychological needs. Investigators are studying the patient's and family's reactions to the disease, sexual concerns, employment and insurance needs and ways to provide support in these areas.

There are over five million Americans alive today who have a history of cancer, and three million were diagnosed five or more years ago. Most can be considered cured—that is, they have no evidence of the disease and have the same life expectancy as a person who never had cancer. Others can expect to be saved by earlier diagnosis and prompt treatment. Except for lung cancer, the survival rates for all forms of the disease are on the increase. For localized breast cancer that is non-invasive (in situ), the survival rate approaches one hundred percent.[137]

Progress has been made in the early diagnosis and treatment of breast cancer. In the future, the search will continue for newer and better ways to treat or prevent the disease. The following developments indicate the directions of current and future research.

BENEFITS OF EARLY DETECTION

The time to detect cancer is *early,* when it is treatable. In their joint Breast Cancer Detection Demonstration Program, the American Cancer Society and National Cancer Institute found that mammography—low-dose x-ray examination—could find cancers so small that they could not be felt by even the most experienced examiner. Other experiments using sound waves, infrared, computers, and electromagnets offer the hope that one day even the smallest cancers will be identified and treated before they get out of control.

Research is also being directed toward other detection devices that do not use radiation at all. The same high-energy sound waves used to destroy kidney stones, for example, may prove to be a new way to detect and treat breast cancer. Techniques such as thermography (infrared heat patterns) and computerized tomography to show more accurately a tumor's shape and location are being studied for their possible effectiveness and appropriate use.

Perhaps the most revolutionary new detection device is nuclear magnetic resonance (NMR) which uses a huge electromagnet to detect tumors by sensing the vibrations of the different atoms in the body. It also permits detailed study of cell physiology, which can help us to eventually determine just why the cancer cell goes haywire and how the body's immune system does and does not react to it. Recent studies of proteins in the blood and how so-called cancer genes (oncogenes) work may provide doctors with new methods of diagnosing early cancers.

Clearly, thousands of lives could be saved each year through early detection not only of breast cancer but cancers of the cervix, uterus, and colon, which offer the greatest opportunity for treatment and cure. For this reason, it is most important to persuade more women to practice monthly breast self-examination, have mammograms or other medical tests, and become familiar with the accepted guidelines for the early detection of cancer.

THE FUTURE OF BREAST SURGERY

Operations used in the surgical treatment of breast cancer have undergone dramatic changes during the past one hundred years. The radical treatment of breast cancer is used infrequently (3%) and conservation surgical techniques are now in vogue since the results are quite similar in survival.

Improvements in surgical techniques and "staging" of the disease have made possible more conservative management of early cancers. This has meant in the case of early minimal breast cancers that many patients have been able to retain all or part of the breast. For others, advances in reconstructive surgery using skin-muscle grafts or implants has become an important rehabilitation choice for women who have had a mastectomy.

Surgical equipment is being improved also. An easy to use surgical knife, which can be harnessed to microwaves to "cook" or cauterize wounds at the same moment an incision is made is considered helpful. This technique has the advantage of closing the blood vessels and lymphatics as the tissue is cut. A laser knife is also being used to treat areas in the body so as not to damage surrounding healthy tissue. Freezing tumors with extreme cold (cryosurgery) is another method of destroying tumors.

All women should realize, however, that conservative or limited surgery (lumpectomy or quadrectomy) will not become the treatment of choice for all breast cancers even in the future. The reason for this is that a large number of breast cancers are detected in the advanced or invasive stage when limited surgery is neither effective nor practical. This may change as more tumors are detected in the earlier noninvasive stage and we learn more about the long-term results of such conservation operations. Right now, the operation most frequently done on breast cancer is the modified mastectomy which is less disfiguring and disabling than radical mastectomy. Many of these women have reconstructive surgery done after the mastectomy.

RADIATION

Intraoperative radiation is being studied as a way to give x-ray treatment at the time of surgery for breast cancer and colon cancer, with the idea being to eliminate residual cancer cells. There's little evidence, however, that such treatment during or following limited surgery—lumpectomy, for example—works effectively on every patient. (See Chapter 9) The problem is that radiation treatment has delayed damaging effects that sometimes take fifteen to twenty years to show up and radiation therapy itself can produce a cancer.

For patients who do undergo radiation therapy, frequent scanning by computerized tomography may enable the radiologist to pinpoint the tumor more precisely in order to provide more accurate radiation dosage while sparing normal tissue. This is the subject of several recent studies and the results are being put into clinical use at many large hospitals. Elsewhere, researchers are trying to develop a special brassiere that contains sensors to pick up hot spots in breast tissue that could signal a malignancy, and radioactive implants have been used in women recovering from a lumpectomy to destroy any residual cancer cells.

CHEMOTHERAPY

Chemotherapy has not been completely successful in preventing the recurrence of breast cancer or preventing spread. The concept of the additive use of chemotherapy, has been a good one, however, to attempt to interfere in different ways with the rapid cell division and growth of the cancer cell.

Many patients with breast cancer are now being treated successfully with combination chemotherapy, with cytotoxic drugs and hormones to shrink advanced tumors or bring about a remission. There is no doubt that they are extremely helpful in the palliation of the breast cancer patient who has recurrence or metastatic disease.

The next step is to see if these and other agents can reduce cancer in high-risk patients by interrupting the process in which different kinds of substances, known as initiators and promotors, cause the cancer to develop and spread. Unusual infections, common in cancer patients, may also be better controlled by new understanding of antibiotic treatment and antibodies.

There's even evidence that the time of day anticancer drugs are administered may make a difference in increasing their effectiveness and minimizing their undesirable side effects, such as hair loss, mouth sores, digestive upsets and skin rashes. This can be devastating to patients. Doctors must maintain a delicate balance between dose and frequency to ameliorate or eliminate such side effects. These studies indicate that successful chemotherapy may be best achieved by timing drugs to when they are best tolerated by the patient. About fifty drugs have been found effective against cancer, and others that are still being tested hold promise.

IMMUNOTHERAPY

Surgery, chemotherapy, and radiation or a combination of all, so far has failed to come up with a consistent cure for breast cancer.

I have always thought the immune system and how it works is the most important aspect in attempting to control breast cancer. Anyone who has treated large numbers of breast cancer patients has noted how variable the body's response is in different individuals. Some patients have a small breast cancer and no matter how you treat them, the cancer is relentless and the patient succumbs in a short period of time. Others have large cancers with advanced disease and yet their alarm system (immune system) is able to respond and they live a useful and healthy life.

Our research scientists have just begun to unlock the method by which the immune system functions. I will project that a few things will develop. Once we isolate the intimidating factor in breast cancer (virus, chemicals, hormones, or their combinations, etc.) we should be able to isolate the factors that react to fight the cancer. These factors should then be able to be grown in genetic factories and used to enhance the body's immune system response. The possibility of developing a vaccine is not as far fetched as some people think, particularly for those individuals in the high-risk group.

Our basic cancer researchers have already developed ways to strengthen the immune system experimentally by getting more natural killer cells into action to destroy some cancers. Lymphokines, a type of white blood cell is produced in response to an attack of cancer cells on the human body. They go about alerting the immune system to function and to fight the invaders. We are just beginning to learn more about lymphokines and tumor necrosis factors which destroy cancer cells and leave normal cells untouched. As we learn more, their use will become more valuable.

CAN CANCER BE PREVENTED?

Chemoprevention studies with agents like synthetic retinoids (cousins of vitamin A), beta-carotene, folic acid and other vitamins and minerals are being undertaken to see if they can prevent cancer. Studies of dietary intervention are examining the effect of low-fat diets in women with breast cancer. The risk for breast, uterine and colon cancers increases for obese women so this is a worthy area of investigation. Foods rich in vitamin A and C may help lower the risk for cancers of the breast and colon.

Extensive research is under way to evaluate and clarify the role of diet and nutrition in the development of cancer. At this point, no direct cause-and-effect relationship has been proven, though several studies show that some foods may increase or decrease the risks for certain types of cancer (Chapter 10). Evidence indicates that women might reduce their breast cancer risk by eating more cruciferous vegetables (cabbage, broccoli), foods rich in vitamin A and C (carrots, oranges), and low-fat acidophilus milk, which may prevent breast cancer by limiting estrogen circulation and carcinogen-generating enzymes.

Unproven methods of cancer prevention or treatment are bound to surface in the future as they have in the past, and they should be evaluated carefully by patients and doctors alike. A list of ingredients is mandatory on most food and drug products, so the best advice is to read all the labeling carefully.

SUMMARY

Until 100 years ago, medicine was practiced as an art. The physician used his eyes, ears, and hands to accumulate data and information.

Today, with sophisticated machines, we are able to penetrate the human body and outline its anatomical structures. X-ray machines, CAT scans (computed axial tomography) and ultrasound (use of sound waves) are able to visualize pre-selected slices of the human body. Using computer reconstruction techniques, we are able to get a clearer picture of normal and abnormal structures. This has helped in establishing earlier diagnosis of breast cancer.

Great strides are being made in conquering cancer. Never before has so much money, effort and research been mobilized to combat this powerful foe. Cure rates are moving upward with encouraging rapidity, with that of localized noninvasive breast cancer now approaching one hundred percent. Medical science alone cannot conquer cancer. It may never come near you, but do not count on that. Take steps now to outwit, avoid and fight cancer as you would any other danger lurking about.

Simplified Anatomy of the Breast

If you're like three fourths of American women, you found an excuse not to examine your breasts this month, probably because you didn't know how to examine your breasts, or what to look for or were afraid of what you'd find. Now's your chance to change that pattern: If you don't know how to examine your breasts, ask your family doctor or breast surgeon to show you how to do it properly. If you are in the higher risk group or over the age of thirty-eight years, ask that a mammogram be done. If you have a lump or feel that you have an abnormality, insist that it be done. Make sure that a competent radiologist looks at the x-ray and if you're not happy with the recommendations, get another opinion. There is also free literature given out by the American Cancer Society that shows you how to examine your breasts and you can use the information presented in this book to help you in that examination. (See Chapter 2)

Description of the breasts (See Figure 8)

The breasts, or mammary glands, are made up of soft tissue and glands that are surrounded by fat, which are arranged in a complicated pattern of lobes, somewhat in the form of a wagon wheel. The milk ducts lead into the nipple. There are about twenty-five openings on the nipple that connect to the ducts in an organized pattern so that if a pregnancy occurs, the glands produce milk for the baby's nutrition. Around the areola (the circular area around the nipple) are little glands that enlarge during pregnancy that lubricate the nipple during nursing.

There are many factors that determine the size and shape of the

Figure 8

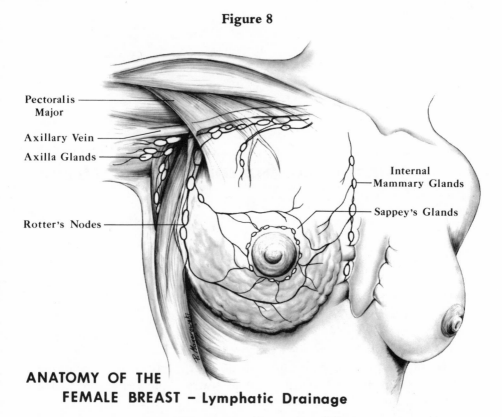

Pectoralis Major

Axillary Vein

Axilla Glands

Rotter's Nodes

Internal Mammary Glands

Sappey's Glands

ANATOMY OF THE
FEMALE BREAST – Lymphatic Drainage

breasts, such as genetics, nutrition, pregnancy, and hormones. Practically all variations in size are normal.

The glandular tissue in the breasts varies with the level of estrogen during the normal monthly cycle, causing the breasts to increase and decrease in size. Fatty tissue fills out the breasts making them round and smooth. The breasts are supported by muscles against the chest wall and ligaments that attach to the ribs, shoulders, clavicle and sternum.

Losing weight will often get rid of some of the fat and make the breasts smaller. Certain exercises, like aerobics, will develop muscles in the vicinity of the breasts, making them seem larger and firmer. Extremely large breasts or too early development of the breasts can be a sign of glandular or other disorder. Breasts may be firm and high or flabby and pendulous. The shape of the breast appears in many cases to be inherited.

The breasts change shape with pregnancy due to the increase in the amount of glandular tissue and the engorgement of the breasts by the production of milk. At the menopause the breasts change shape due to the lack of hormonal stimulation from the ovaries. Women with large breasts sometimes have breast reductions done at this time for cosmetic reasons.

Exercise can sometimes be done to tone up the supporting muscles to help prevent breast sag.

Lymph node drainage from the breast. (See Figure 8)

It is very important for a surgeon or cancer specialist treating breast cancer to know the anatomy of the breast. The doctor should know the blood supply coming into the tissue (arterial) and the blood supply draining the area (venous) and more importantly, know the lymph gland drainage of the breast.

It is also important for the woman to know this because then she can better understand why she checks certain body areas when she does breast self-examination. One area to be checked is the glands under the armpit, because the breast has many lymphatic channels that can carry cancer cells from the breast tissue to the glands and when they become involved a metastases or spread has developed and treatment methods change.

The distribution of the lymphatic drainage of the breast was established by research started many years ago. Mercurial injection techniques were used to demonstrate the rich plexus under the nipple.[138] This is why tumors in this area can go in many different directions when they spread. The main lymphatic collecting trunks lead to the axilla[139] (armpit).

Another lymphatic drainage area passes beneath the chest wall muscles (pectoralis major muscles) and leads to the apex of the axilla (armpit). The lymph glands (nodes) between the pectoralis major and minor muscles are known as Rotter's nodes.[140]

Handley[141] has written an excellent book demonstrating the multiple lymphatic pathways and he has pointed out the importance of the internal mammary chain of lymph nodes and its association with breast cancer.

What all this means is that the primary site of the breast tumor helps determine where the cancer will spread if the cancer gets into the lymphatic channels. The main channels are the axilla (armpit) for lateral site tumors and the internal mammary chain (under the breast bone—sternum) for medial site tumors. One often cannot determine where tumors under the nipple (subareolar) will spread to (Sappey's nodes).

What Does the Tissue Analysis Mean?

There are many factors that determine the outcome of the breast cancer patient: the size of the primary tumor, the type of tumor present on tissue analysis, whether or not the lymph nodes are involved with spread of the cancer, the steroid hormone receptors, if the cancer has gotten into the blood stream and involved the bones or other organs, the menopausal status of the patient, and the patient's own immunity or ability to resist the cancer. Other factors also play a role but these are the important ones.

Staging systems have been devised prior to treatment and have often been found to be inaccurate. Analysis of the tissue, by a pathologist, is still the best method to determine extent of disease.

The importance of the analysis of the tissue removed, the breast tumor and the glands under the armpit cannot be over-emphasized. For it is the proper analysis of this tissue that will direct the proper treatment to be given if further treatment is necessary. The single most important factor in relationship to prognosis is whether the axillary lymph nodes are involved with cancer or not.

When the lump is removed from the breast by the surgeon a frozen section or immediate microscopic study of the tissue is done. If the tumor is cancerous on frozen section, that tissue will be saved for a complex analysis and special staining of the cells to establish exactly what type of malignant breast tumor is present.

Part of the tissue will be saved to determine its estrogen and pro-gesterone (female hormones) content. This allows the doctor to deter-mine if he is dealing with a hormone dependent tumor or not and the information is valuable to be documented so that if spread of the tumor occurs (metastases) later on, hormonal manipulation and/or chemotherapy can be used to improve survival and the quality of life of the patient.

A few years ago, hormone manipulation was always done with surgery by removing the ovaries and/or the adrenal glands, which are where most of the estrogen hormones are made. Since the majority of breast cancers are estrogen dependent, it was rationalized that by removing the source of estrogen, the tumor growth would be stopped and survival time would be increased. This is exactly what happened.

Basic researchers working with pharmaceutical drug companies then developed estrogen blocking agents (Tamoxifen) which worked just as well as the ablative surgery.

This is why if you have a biopsy of a breast tumor that is diagnosed as cancer you should ask your doctor whether the tumor tissue has been sent for analysis of its estrogen and progesterone hormonal levels.

TUMOR MARKERS

A search for a specific tumor marker for breast cancer has been going on for many years. An attempt to find a substance that can be measured quantitatively by biochemical or immunochemical means has been unsuccessful so far. If one could find a breast cancer tumor marker, one could screen large female population groups or groups of females that are known to be in the high risk group and detect the cancer at an early stage and hopefully treat it before regional or systemic metastases occur.

Tumor markers can be enzymes, hormones, specific proteins, metabolites or tumor antigens. Unfortunately, the tumor markers are not good in early breast cancer but have been helpful in the patient with breast cancer that is disseminated. *CEA antigen,* which is a tumor marker, has been used to follow patients with colon cancer and is now being used to follow the course of the breast cancer patient with diffuse metastases. Some tumor markers (CEA) can be elevated with boney metastases in addition to liver metastases.

Estrogen and Progesterone Receptors

Estrogen and progesterone receptors are proteins in the tumor tissue and the best time to obtain and analyze these receptors is when the biopsy of the breast tumor is done.

In order to have proper evaluation of steroid hormone receptors, the surgeon has to do his job right when he does the biopsy, the pathologist must properly freeze and care for the specimen and the laboratory accurately assess the material.

Steroid hormone receptor tissue assays (estrogen and progesterone) are important at the present time, because they allow the doctor to select therapy that may be helpful in treatment for recurrent or systemic metastases.

The effectiveness of endocrine therapy closely correlates with the measured hormone receptor levels. Hormone manipulation seems to benefit the postmenopausal patient the best. Women who develop recurrent disease after the menopause and have positive axillary nodes live longer free of disease with hormone blocking agents such as Tamoxifen if they have hormone receptor positive tumors.

What lumps need to be biopsied?

The majority of lumps or thickenings in the breast are benign and do not need to be biopsied. Now that sophisticated imaging devices, such as mammography, are available to the cancer specialist, fewer women need a sampling of the tissue. Mammography is about ninety percent accurate in predicting cancers. If there is any doubt about whether a biopsy should be done or not, the clinical judgment of the surgeon should prevail.

Women who are young and actively menstruating have many changes in the breast during their cycle. Some of these changes are altered by the birth control pill.

Various inflammations of the breast (mastitis) are quite common. They may follow childbirth or injury and often become chronic and can be confused with cancer. They are usually not serious, although they can be very painful especially before the menstrual periods.

Breast lumps can develop during pregnancy and usually are benign. However, cancer can also develop so that the pregnant woman should continue to check her breasts during pregnancy.

Cysts and other swellings occur fairly frequently in the breasts and are seldom dangerous; usually they are drained with a needle in the doctor's office and that's the end of it. Abscesses may result from infection and can be drained or treated with antibiotics.

Most cancers of the breast are firm and solid and increase in size. They are usually picked up by breast self-examination or are found by screening methods on the x-ray picture.

If the tissue removed is questionable as to whether it is cancerous or not, then an unbiased consultation with another medical center pathologist should be obtained.

The Armed Forces Institute of Pathology in Washington, D.C. maintains a diagnostic center to aid hospitals in obtaining a proper tissue diagnosis and these second opinions concerning the tissue removed can be obtained by the patient. This is recommended however, only where there is a difficulty in establishing a diagnosis. This is not recommended for the routine breast cancer case.

Axillary lymph nodes - glandular spread

The removal of the lymph glands under the armpit (axillary lymph nodes) after the diagnosis of breast cancer has been established by biopsy is the single most important procedure done to determine how well the patient is going to do.

The number of lymph nodes involved is used to determine what type of treatment should be given. This is why it is extremely important that a good adequate axillary dissection be done in all breast cancer cases even if a lumpectomy is the treatment selected so the breast can be saved.

Doing an axillary dissection stages the disease and the examination of the lymph gland tissue tells the doctor whether the tumor has spread or not. In other words, a full axillary dissection should be done and not just a sampling of nodes.

Clinical staging is inaccurate and research studies using this method are not factual. The inaccuracy of examination of the armpit by palpation for spread of tumor to the axilla has been established.

An Attempt to Define Cancer

Cancer was named by Hippocrates, the father of medicine. The Greek word is *karkinos* or crab, and Hippocrates named it that because of the pincer-like projections he noticed when examining women with breast cancer. Of course, by the time the disease appeared in this form, it was almost always fatal. As a result, doctors in ancient times thought cancer incurable. Today we know differently.

It is not known why certain women get breast cancer and others do not. Genetic, lifestyle and environmental factors seem involved—recent studies show that women who eat a diet rich in fatty foods are more prone to this type of cancer. Obesity also appears to be a risk factor, as well as hormones and stress. What we do know is that cancer is a large group of diseases characterized by uncontrolled growth and spread of abnormal or malignant cells. Moreover, it is important to recognize that breast cancer often is curable if diagnosed early.

What is a cancer cell?

The human body is made up of millions of cells that combine to form tissues and organs with specific functions to enable the organism to survive and adapt in a changing environment. The normal healthy cell has a specific site it functions at. It requires water, food, and oxygen to survive and is capable of duplication and reproduction.

The cancer cell varies from the normal healthy cell. It has a marked diversity in regards to reproduction and morphology. The cell surface or membrane is different; it is able to invade tissues and organs and destroy them. It has abnormal growth rates and can spread to distant organs attaching itself to form new cancers.

Both the normal cell and the cancer cell have a control mechanism or nucleus inside the cell. The cancer cell is different in that it is able to multiply more rapidly. The control center of the cell or nucleus is often divided or in the process of dividing. If there are many abnormal cells like this seen under the microscope the diagnosis of cancer is made.

What causes the normal cell to become a cancer cell and go haywire is still unknown. Is it due to a virus and if so, how does the virus penetrate the normal cell membrane and get at the control center (the nucleus) that controls the cell's action?

Or is the cancer cell a cancer cell from the beginning? Is it a mutant that has been developed by environmental effects upon the cell, such as chemicals, nutrients, or adverse oxygenation effects?

We know that the cell has a membrane and that nutrients and chemicals diffuse in and out of the cell through the membrane. The cancer cell interacts with the normal healthy cell and therefore, in order to penetrate or spread, the cell membrane is important. The ability of the cancer cell membrane to stick (become adhesive) or not stick to a blood vessel wall determines the capability of the cancer cell to metastasize or spread.

Not all cancer cells metastasize. Why some spread and others do not is difficult to determine. The cancer cells or clumps of cells can break off (tumor emboli) and get into the lymphatics (nodes or glands) or into the blood stream.

As a tumor grows in size, not all cells within the tumor are actively dividing and as the tumor continues to grow and get larger, the percentage of actively dividing cells may decrease. This may be due to nutrition (blood supply) or other factors such as hormones or to the human body's own defense mechanism attempting to slow down the growth of the tumor (the immune system).

Tumors have a rate of growth that can be measured. This is called the doubling time of the tumor. This is the time the cancer cell takes to reproduce itself. The range of doubling time can vary immensely from one week to two years or much longer. For example, the typical breast cancer usually requires two years to reach a size of one-half inch.

THE WAY CANCER SPREADS

Local Invasion

Cancer cells can invade and destroy local tissues. If local invasion occurs and the cancer is in an area of the body that can be surgically removed without endangering the patient (the host) surgery can control the cancer. Radiation can control the smaller cancers if distant spread has not occurred.

An example of a tumor that invades locally is a skin cancer (basal cell) that often occurs on the exposed areas of the body and is related to prolonged exposure to sunlight (radiation). Excellent treatment results can be attained by surgery or radiation.

However, in contrast to skin cancers, local cancer invasion can be lethal if the tumor develops in an area of the body that cannot be easily resected surgically or treated by other methods. For example, esophageal cancer (the esophagus is the feeding tube from mouth to stomach and is located in an area of the body that cannot be easily removed). The heart and breathing tubes that go to the lungs are right next to the esophagus making it more difficult to treat this area.

Certain brain tumors are another example of how local invasion can destroy the host and because of their location they rarely spread outside of the skull. These tumors are very difficult to treat.

Metastases

If the cancer specialist could prevent metastases (spread) from occurring, most cancers could be cured by controlling the primary tumor if it occurs at a site that can be adequately treated.

Once the cell or cells have broken off from the primary tumor the cells flow to glands or distant organs usually thru lymphatics or vascular channels. Osmotic pressures or mobility of the cells (movement) aid the flow.

Cancer cells have the ability to adhere together to form a clump of cells or metastasize at the distant site and this probably has something to do with the complex mechanism of clotting of blood.[142] A certain concentration of cancer cells has to be present in order to get a take (metastases) at a distant site. It has been known for years that migratory thrombophlebitis can be associated with diffuse overwhelming cancer;[143] pancreatic cancer for instance.

The total mechanism by which blood clots or does not clot when patients have cancer is unclear. The hypercoagulable state associated with cancer probably has something to do with thrombin (an enzyme that participates in the clotting of blood) and the venous vessel wall and breakdown products of the necrotic tumor.

Migratory thrombophlebitis is resistant to routine anticoagulant therapy and may appear months or years before cancer develops. The human body's mechanism by which blood remains liquid is unclear to the scientist. There are many factors in the vascular spaces which prevent blood from clotting, such as fibrinolytic enzymes and numerous other factors.

Attempts have been made to prevent metastases by giving blood thinners such as heparin and dicumerol and this has been successful in preventing metastases or a take in the experimental animal.[144] It has not been successful in humans.

Cancer cells have other interesting characteristics which should be mentioned in regards to metastasis. Once the clump of cancer cells or metastasis has anchored at a distant site (usually in the capillary beds) neovascularization of the tumor occurs. By neovascularization is meant, the growth of new blood vessels as the tumor gets larger. The rate of growth of the lining of the blood vessels feeding the tumor (the endothelium) might have something to do with the actual size of the tumor.

The properties of the vessel wall (endothelium) are extremely important, for if the vessel wall is damaged, the clotting mechanism (coagulation process) goes on more rapidly, particularly in the small vessels on the surface, or smaller peripheral vessels in organs. It is here that the rate of flow is lower and the exchange of nutrients and chemicals through cell membranes occurs.

Not all cancer cells or clumps of cells that break off from the primary tumor are capable of a take at a distant site (metastasis). In fact, very few actually survive. This may be related to the inability to attach to the vessel or the cohesiveness of the cancer cell or to host resistance.[145]

Once the cancer cell or clumps of cells get free, the immune mechanism of the human body comes into play. The ability of one human body to destroy circulating cancer cells and another to allow it to take or metastasize relates to the immune mechanism.

Immune mechanism

The ability of the body to inhibit or attempt to destroy cancer cells before they spread makes up part of the immune mechanism. The immune mechanism works in several different ways, not all of which are fully understood. Basically, certain types of white blood cells are alerted to the presence of invading cancer cells and form antibodies to fight and destroy the invaders. This can be seen graphically in the rejection of donor tissue or organs during transplant operations, and is the subject of much current cancer research.

Man-made antibodies such as hybridomas (antibody factories) and highly specific monoclonal antibodies, for example, can be produced that will recognize cancer cells only, and thus be able to detect cancer early, when the disease is most curable. Monoclonal antibodies already have been used to deliver drugs directly to tumors, killing them but sparing healthy tissue. Gene splicing has produced interferon, which may ultimately be valued not so much for itself, as for its role in heralding a whole new class of compounds called "biologic response modifiers," which will fight cancer by stimulating the body's immune system.

As we increase our knowledge of the immune system and how it works, we can expect genetic engineering to find other ways to fight cancer as well. Investigators are already looking for ways to detect cancer earlier by tracing a cell's biochemical markers. They are exploring evidence that certain organs or parts of the body are more involved than others perhaps because of a breakdown in the individual's immune system. They're testing the hypothesis that certain chemicals or environments enhance the body's receptivity to cancer.

Epidemiologists know, for example, that cancer affects people in some parts of the world more than others and that breast cancer is more common in obese women who eat fatty foods than in thinner women whose diet is high in fish and protein. They point to the high incidence of cervical cancer among women who are sexually active, and to the increased rates of lung cancer among women smokers. Other clues are being pursued by researchers in the substances or lifestyles that seem to serve as defense mechanisms against cancer.

Fortunately, cancer is not contagious, or is it? Recently the disease entity *AIDS* which can be transmitted sexually by homosexuals or thru the blood, was found to produce Kaposi's Sarcoma, a form of cancer. It is perhaps one of the few types of cancers that can be transmitted by a virus. Practically all cancers are not contagious, however. Most cancers are not transmitted from one individual to another.

Selection of site of metastases

There also seems to be a selective process by the cancer cell or clump of cells (metastases) as to where it wants to live and grow. Specific organs seem to be the target site for metastases: these sites can be predicted in certain cancers. Certain organs are not often involved with metastatic disease. Is it that the ground is not fertile there for the cancer seed or seeds to grow?[146] Or does that organ contain anti-cancer substances?[147] An example is the spleen which is not often involved with metastatic cancer and yet if an overwhelming infection in the body occurs, the spleen frequently shows evidence of the infection. How often has one seen the bones of the hands or feet involved with metastatic cancer and yet in breast cancer the other bones of the body are frequently involved.

When a patient gets more than one cancer there seems to be a specific site that the second cancer will develop in. It usually develops in a predictable site and tissue. In other words, there seems to be a tissue specificity when more than one cancer develops.[148]

Factors that produce cancers

The exogenous factors that produce cancer are too numerous to mention. Just a few important ones that we see in our daily lives are: Radiation from the sun producing skin cancers such as basal cell cancer. Radiation probably plays a role in activating the lethal pigmented melanoma of the skin. Evidence that viruses are being incriminated in more and more different types of cancer appear every day in research. Leukemias (blood cancer) and lymphoma (glandular cancer) show clustering of the disease in many areas of the world.

The acquired immune deficiency syndrome, seen in homosexuals, Haitians and can be transmitted by blood transfusions produced a cancerous tumor, Kaposi's Sarcoma, in all likelihood caused by a virus. This disease has allowed the scientific community to have a human model to study the role of viral infections in relation to causative factors, the immune system and the production of a deadly cancer.

Other viruses have been incriminated in precancerous and invasive cancers of the cervix and these may be sexually transmitted.[149]

A human papillomavirus (HPU) has been isolated and can produce tumors of the esophagus and has also been linked to squamous cell cancer in other body areas.[150] This virus which is acquired either congenitally or through sexual transmission may be increasing because of the apparent growing prevalence of oral genital sexual intercourse.

Nutritional factors, the food we eat and the water we drink are extremely important factors to consider in producing cancer and *preventing cancer*. Natural foods and specific foods that can be helpful in one's diet such as citrus fruits and foods with specific high concentrations of vitamins such as A and C have been written about extensively. Food additives to preserve food and coloring or flavoring to make food appear better have been *incriminated* in producing cancer.

Pesticides and chemical wastes from industrial plants that get into our drinking water can trigger a cancer in the human host and workers that worked in asbestos plants, that were not properly protected, invariably developed debilitating lung disease and cancer.

Does age play a role in producing cancer?

As the body ages, or its parts start to wear out, is the immune response capable of handling the invasion by cancer? Only a small number of cancers occur in the younger age group and many of these may be related to genetic factors. The stress of living in today's society has its toll and contributes to the aging process.

Stress and the immune system are interrelated. Most cancers occur in the fourth, fifth, and sixth decades of life. Age certainly is a factor in the development of breast cancer.

In my practice, ninety percent of the breast cancers developed after the age of thirty-eight years. Only ten percent occurred in the younger age group. Most breast cancers develop at or shortly after the menopause. With the aging process, the body's tissues and cells start to wear out. The inability to respond makes the woman more susceptible to cancer.

As our basic science researchers unlock the mechanisms of the immune system, we should be able to find the key to a cure for breast cancer in the future.

Does Your Personality Make You Cancer Prone?

Which comes first, the chicken or the egg? Do you have a specific personality that makes you more susceptible to get cancer and then you get cancer, or do you get cancer and then develop the personality change? There is no concrete evidence that your personality predisposes you to get cancer, although there is positive evidence that exogenous forces, those that we live in around us, may play a big part in whether we get cancer.

This book has discussed many of these exogenous forces. The *water you drink,* which may contain hazardous waste that produces leukemia; the *food you eat,* which may contain excessive animal fats or contain harmful preservatives that can cause colon and possibly breast cancer; and the *the air you breathe,* which may fill your lungs with pollution or smoking, and produce lung cancer.

There are other subtle forces that have a strong effect on the development of one's personality. Your parents, teachers, and peers apply their own personal attitudes upon you as you grow up and once you get older and your personality becomes more fixed, your ability to adapt to stress may have something to do with that up-bringing. Cancer occurs most often in the older age group, the fifth and sixth decades of life when it is more difficult to change one's personality.

In today's society, everyone lives with some degree of stress and one's response and adaptation determines their quality of life and how they survive and whether they will survive.

We know for instance, that individuals in high stress positions are more prone to get stomach ulcers, bowel changes, such as diarrhea or constipation and even heart attacks. Police, with hypertension and potential heart disease, are an example and in some states are disability compensated and retired.

Some of these people have been classified as Type A personalities and they are supposedly more likely to have heart attacks.

Irritable bowel syndrome, which is seen frequently in women, is influenced by psychosocial factors and causes diarrhea and constipation. The spastic colon effect seems to happen most often in the over-anxious individual. These people seem to be more concerned and preoccupied with what is happening in the outside world.

The psychosomatic aspects of certain diseases are almost irrefutable and there are some suggested disease patterns that predispose the individual to get cancer such as ulcerative colitis that often goes on to cause cancer of the colon. Prolonged excessive smoking goes on to cause cancer of the lung, yet not all heavy smokers get lung cancer. Is there a certain type of personality that is more prone to get that type of cancer?

When you talk to smokers and try to convince them to stop, their reply is that they can't. "I'm dependent on smoking. I release my tension this way. It keeps my weight down. If I stop smoking I eat too much and become fat." There is no doubt that, in some cases, smoking is associated with a dependent type personality.

Excessive alcoholic intake is a known causative factor in esophageal cancer and specific character disorders have been associated with this problem. The compulsive drinker is usually a lonely, depressed individual who is more introverted, more withdrawn, and less aggressive.

Personality and Breast Cancer

Many studies have been done on breast cancer patients to try to determine specific personality traits that might be associated with the development of the disease. In my practice I have noted that there is no one specific personality that causes women to develop breast cancer and that women with all personality types may develop the disease.

In the long period of time that I have been taking care of breast cancer patients, I have noticed that most of these women become immediately depressed once the diagnosis has been made. Their anxiety increases and in many cases there is a guilt feeling and an extreme element of hostility—Why did it happen to me?

Part of this depression may be related to the fear that they may need a mastectomy or that they may die. The stress associated with the diagnosis of breast cancer is quite evident. Is it possible that stress itself preceded the development of the cancer and made the woman more vulnerable to get the disease?

In a questionnaire, sent to my patients, over forty percent with operable breast cancer stated that they had either an acute stress (6 mos.) or chronic stress (5 yrs.) situation prior to getting their breast cancer. An example of an acute stress was usually the loss of a loved one (death in the family). A chronic stress was living with an unemployed alcoholic for a long period of time.

The normal physiological mechanisms that are disturbed by the psychological input such as acute or chronic stress has a big toll on our bodies and as to how this functions, thru the immune or hormonal systems is beginning to be investigated and documented. (See Chapter 11—Stress and the Immune System)

Acute and chronic stress has an effect on our immune system and actual blood changes have been documented with effects on the T cells and B cells. The immune system can become depressed and this can make the individual more susceptible to getting any type of cancer.

Personal appearance and diet are inter-related and how we look is an expression of our personality. Over fifty percent of my patients stated that they were overweight or obese prior to the diagnosis of breast cancer. One can ask the question: Were they under severe stress and then ate excessively to try to compensate in this manner? What effect did the obesity have on their personalities? Did they become more withdrawn and seclusive?

Post-Mastectomy Personality Change

The attitude of the woman following her treatment such as mastectomy for breast cancer, plays a role in how long she will survive and there is a difference in attitudes of the short and long term survivor. The psychosocial aspects following mastectomy are quite complicated and some are discussed in Chapter 14. Some of the answers to the questionnaire that I sent out to all of my breast cancer patients are included in that chapter.

Summary

I'll ask the question again. Which came first, the chicken or the egg? Is there a certain type of personality that predisposes one to get cancer, or does the cancer come first and the personality change follow? I believe that both factors play a role in the etiology and understanding of breast cancer.

Sources for Further Information and Help

Breast Self-Examination

American Cancer Society
4 West 35th Street
New York, NY 10001
Phone: 212-736-3030

American Medical Association
535 North Dearborn Street
Chicago, IL 60610

Cancer Information Center
National Cancer Institute
Bethesda, MD 20205
Phone: 800-422-6237

Consumer Information Center
U.S. Government Printing
  Office
Pueblo, CO 81009

Comprehensive Cancer Centers

Univ. of Alabama in
  Birmingham Comprehensive
  Cancer Center

Lurleen Wallace Tumor Institute
1824 6th Ave. S.
Birmingham, AL 35294
Phone: 205-934-5077

Univ. of Southern California
Comprehensive Cancer Center
1441 Eastlake Ave.
Los Angeles, CA 90033
Phone: 213-224-6416

UCLA-Jonsson Comprehensive
  Cancer Center
Louis Factor Health Sciences
  Bldg.
10833 LeConte Ave.
Los Angeles, CA 90024
Phone: 213-825-5268

Yale Comprehensive Cancer
  Center
Yale Univ. School of Medicine
333 Cedar Street
New Haven, CT 06510
Phone: 203-785-4095

Georgetown Univ./Howard Univ. Comprehensive Cancer Center
Washington, DC

Comprehensive Cancer Center for the State of Florida
Univ. of Miami School of Medicine
1475 N.W. 12th Avenue
Miami, FL 33101
Phone: 305-545-7707

Illinois Cancer Council
36 S. Wabash Ave.
Chicago, IL 60603
Phone: 312-346-9813

Johns Hopkins Oncology Center
600 North Wolfe Street
Baltimore, MD 21205
Phone: 301-955-8822

Dana-Farber Cancer Institute
44 Binney Street
Boston, MA 02115
Phone: 617-732-3555

Michigan Cancer Foundation
Meyer L. Prentis Cancer Center
110 East Warren Ave.
Detroit, MI 48201
Phone: 313-833-0710

Mayo Clinic
200 First Street, S.W.
Rochester, MN 55905
Phone: 507-284-8964

Columbia Univ. Cancer Research Center
701 W. 168th St.
New York, NY 10032
Phone: 212-694-3647

Memorial Sloan-Kettering Cancer Ctr.
1275 York Avenue
New York, NY 10021
Phone: 212-794-6561

Roswell Park Memorial Institute
666 Elm Street
Buffalo, NY 14263
Phone: 716-845-5770

Duke Comprehensive Cancer Center
P.O. Box 3814
Duke University Medical Center
Durham, NC 27710
Phone: 919-684-2282

Ohio State University Comprehensive Cancer Center
410 West 12th Avenue
Columbus, OH 43210
Phone: 614-422-5022

Fox Chase/ University of Pennsylvania Cancer Center
Philadelphia, PA

The Univ. of Texas System Cancer Center
M.D. Anderson Hospital and Tumor Institute
6723 Bertner Avenue
Houston, TX 77030
Phone: 713-792-6000

Fred Hutchinson Cancer Research Ctr.
1124 Columbia Street
Seattle, WA 98104
Phone: 206-292-2930

Wisconsin Clinical Cancer Center

University of Wisconsin
600 Highland Avenue
Madison, WI 53792
Phone: 608-263-8610

Drugs and Radiation

Food and Drug Administration
5600 Fishers Lane
Rockville, MD 20857
Phone: 202-872-0382

Medisense
1133 Avenue of the Americas
New York, NY 10036

Patient's Medical Library
20 Hospital Drive
Toms River, NJ 08753
Phone: 800-222-0077

Public and Professional Affairs
U.S. Pharmacopeia
12601 Twinbrook Parkway
Rockville, MD 20852

Food and Nutrition

American Council on Science
and Health
47 Maple Street
Summit, NJ 07901

American Institute for Cancer
Research
Washington, DC 20069

American Institute of Nutrition
9650 Rockville Pike
Bethesda, MD 20014

Center for Science in the Public
Interest
1755 S Street, N.W.
Washington, DC 20009

Consumer Food Safety
Department of Agriculture
Washington, DC 20250
Phone: 202-472-4485

Food Safety Council
1725 K Street, N.W.
Washington, DC 20006

Gynecology and Obstetrics

American College of
Obstetricians and
Gynecologists
600 Maryland Ave., S.W.
Washington, DC 20024
Phone: 202-638-5577

Center for Reproductive and
Sexual Health
424 East 62nd Street
New York, NY 10021

National Women's Health
Network
224 Seventh Street, S.E.
Washington, DC 20003
Phone: 202-543-9222

Planetree Health Resource Center
2040 Webster Street
San Francisco, CA 94115
Phone: 415-346-4636

Public Health

American Public Health Assoc.
1015 15th Street, N.W.
Washington, DC 20005

Center for Medical Consumers
237 Thompson Street
New York, NY 10012
Phone: 212-674-7105

Consumer Health Information
  Center
680 East 600 South
Salt Lake City, UT 84103
Phone: 801-364-9318

National Health Information
  Clearinghouse
U.S. Public Health Service
Washington, DC 20013
Phone: 800-336-4797

Personal Health Record
Metropolitan Life Ins. Co.
One Madison Avenue
New York, NY 10010

President's Council on Physical
  Fitness
450 5th Street, N.W.
Washington, DC 20001

Public Citizen Health Research
  Group
200 P Street, N.W.
Washington, DC 20036
Phone: 202-872-0382

World Health Organization
Room 2427
United Nations, NY 10017

Rehabilitation and Counseling

American Family Therapy
  Assoc.
15 Bond Street
Great Neck, NY 11021

Breast Cancer Advisory Center
Box 224
Kensington, MD 20795

Cancer Counseling and Research
  Ctr.

1300 Summit Avenue
Fort Worth, TX 76102
Phone: 817-335-4823

Family Service Assoc. of
  America
44 East 23rd Street
New York, NY 10010

Mental Health Clearinghouse
5600 Fishers Lane
Rockville, MD 20857
Phone: 202-443-4513

National Genetics Foundation
55 West 57th Street
New York, NY 10019

National Self-Help
  Clearinghouse
33 West 42nd Street
New York, NY 10036
Phone: 212-840-7606

Reach to Recovery
American Cancer Society
4 West 34th Street
New York, NY 10001
Phone: 212-736-3030

Surgery and Reconstruction

American College of Surgeons
55 East Erie Street
Chicago, IL

American Society of Plastic and
  Reconstructive Surgeons
233 North Michigan Avenue
Chicago, IL 60601

American Surgical Association
32 Fruit Street
Boston, MA 02114

Association of American
  Physicians and Surgeons
8991 Cotswold Drive
Burke, VA 22015

Coalition for the Medical Rights
  of Women
1638 Haight Street
San Francisco, CA 94117

Second Surgical Opinion Hotline
Health and Human Services
Phone: 800-638-6833

Miscellaneous

Encore Program
YWCA

726 Broadway
New York, NY 10003

National Center for Health
  Statistics
3700 East-West Highway
Hyattsville, MD 20782
Phone: 301-436-7085

National Institutes of Health
9000 Rockville Pike
Bethesda, MD 20892

Health and Human Services
  Department
3700 East-West Highway
Hyattsville, MD 20782
Phone: 301-436-6716

Guide to Medical Terms

Adenoma A glandlike growth, usually a benign tumor. If malignant, it is called adenocarcinoma.

Adrenal gland A small gland located just above the kidney. Its secretions (ex. cortisone, adrenalin, aldosterone) affect the functions of other glands and organs in many important ways.

Aesthetic values Pertaining to beauty or improvement of appearence.

Amenorrhea Absence or abnormal stoppage of the menstrual cycle (menses).

Androgen A substance, usually a hormone, that produces male characteristics (see Testosterone).

Anticoagulant A drug capable of slowing the clotting of blood (Ex. Heparin, Dicumerol, Coumadin).

Areola A pigmented ring around a central point, such as the nipple of the breast.

Aspiration A technique used to withdraw fluid or tissue through a needle from a breast tumor.

Atypical Irregular, not conforming to type. Cell that is not normal.

Autoimmune disease Disease in which the body is unable to distinguish between foreign invaders and its own tissues so it produces defensive antibodies against itself, often with serious harm.

Axillary dissection Surgical removal of lymph glands along the axillary vein and armpit.

Benign tumor A tumor that is not malignant (does not contain cancer).

Bilateral breast cancer Cancer involving both breasts at the same time (synchronous) or at different times (metachronous).

Biopsy Removal of a piece of tissue to be examined microscopically for diagnosis.

Bloody nipple discharge Discharge from the nipple usually detected on the underclothing and which usually indicates a benign intraductal papilloma. In rare case can be an indication of cancer.

Bone scan The injection of radioisotopes that concentrate in the bones and then are visualized by imaging techniques and pictures which are recorded to determine abnormalities or bone metastases (spread of breast cancer to bone).

Brachial plexus Group of interjoining nerves in the lower neck that extend to axilla and arm.

Breast self-examination (BSE) Examination of the breasts by the woman to detect lumps visually or by palpation.

Calcifications of the breast Minute calcium deposits within the breast (single or clustered) usually detected by imaging (mammography and xeromammography).

Cancer Malignant tumor. An uncontrolled growth of abnormal cells that invade and destroy the surrounding tissues.

Carcinogen A substance that can cause cancer.

Carcinoma in situ A small or minimal cancer that involves the cells on the surface and has not invaded the subcutaneous tissues.

CAT Abbreviation for computerized axial tomography in which a computer is used to analyze multiple x-rays of soft body tissues.

Cauterize To apply an electrical current to tissue to cut, coagulate or destroy it by heating.

CEA antigen blood test (Carcinoembryonic antigen) A nonspecific blood test used to follow breast cancer patients with metastases (spread) to determine whether the treatment method is working or not. Also used in detection and treatment of colon cancer.

Chemoprevention The use of medicine or vitamins as an aid to prevent disease such as cancer.

Chemotherapy The use of drugs or medicine that may be used in cancer treatment that helps destroy cancer cells.

Clock palpation A method of breast self-examination using the numbers on a clock as a reference to localize lumps of any kind.

Cyst of the breast A sac filled with fluid within the breast. This can be clear yellow fluid or blood tinged fluid and can be single or multiple.

Cytology The study of cells.

Cytotoxic Capable of being cytotoxic or poisonous to cells. Types of medicines or drugs that destroy cells.

DES (Diethylstilbestrol) A synthetic estrogen that has been used in the treatment of breast and prostate cancer. It has been associated with cancer of the vagina in the daughters of women given the compound during pregnancy and has recently been associated with an increased risk for breast cancer for mothers who took the drug.

DNA Abbreviation for deoxyribonucleic acid, a chemical in the human cell that is important in controlling heredity.

Doubling time The time required for a cell to duplicate itself and divide. This can apply to the breast cancer cell and has many variables depending upon the type of tumor, the host resistance, and the media in which it attempts to grow.

Duct ectasia Dilatation or widening of the ducts of the breast, often called periductal mastitis or comedomastitis. It can be associated with a nipple discharge and inflammation and can produce fibrosis and retraction of the nipple.

Dysplasia An appearance of cells that are abnormal and have features that suggest cancer but with insufficient positive changes that can be called cancer.

Edema Swelling caused by collection of fluid in tissues.

Embolus A plug or clot of blood or tumor cells within a blood vessel.

Endothelium A thin layer of cells that line the blood and lymph vessels and the chambers of the heart. Endothelial proliferation is considered necessary for tumor growth.

Epithelium Type of cells found in skin and mucous membranes.

Esophagus The tube that conveys food and liquids from the mouth to the stomach. It has a muscular lining that contracts to aid in propulsion and is lined with epithelium that secretes mucus to allow food to pass downward.

Estrogen A group of steroid female sex hormones produced primarily in the ovaries, adrenal gland, placenta, and fat tissues and essential for the development of the sexual organs and secondary sex characteristics. Synthetic estrogen is used in the birth control pills and as replacement therapy following hysterectomy and oophorectomy.

Estrogen receptor A protein that is found in target tissue cells, such as the breast, that is measured when a breast biopsy for cancer is done. The amount of the measurement of estrogen receptor is used as an aid in directing treatment of breast cancer.

Etiology Causes of disease or the study of the causes of disease.

Exogenous factors External factors that are developed and occur outside a living organism and may have a beneficial or harmful effect on that organism.

Exploratory laparotomy A surgical exploration of the abdomen to help determine the cause for life threatening abdominal pain and discomfort (Ex. appendectomy).

Fascia Thin tissues found beneath the skin between and around muscles and other structures.

Fat necrosis The destruction of fat cells usually secondary to trauma (injury) which can cause retraction of the skin or skin changes that can be confused with breast cancer.

FDA Abbreviation for Food and Drug Administration.

Fibroadenoma A fibrous firm tumor that usually occurs in the young female that is almost always benign. It is usually single but can be multiple. Malignant change can develop in a fibroadenoma but is extremely rare.

Fibrocystic disease A condition seen in females usually during their menstrual years that produces fibrosis or scarring and cystic changes in the breast that are felt as lumps. These lumps appear to get larger and smaller during the menstrual cycle. The cystic changes can be single or multiple. The condition can be confused with more serious changes within the breast.

Food additives Substances that are added to food to preserve it, make it appear better, to retard deterioration, or add flavor. Some food additives can be harmful and carcinogenic.

Food cancer blockers Specific types of vegetables and foods that are felt to have the ability to stop or assist in arresting the growth of the cancer cell.

Frozen section—breast A technique of freezing tissue after removing it from the breast, then cutting it into thin sections by the use of a microtone (cryostat) and then staining the tissues and mounting them on a slide and looking at them under the microscope to establish a diagnosis rapidly.

Genetic Pertaining to the origin or the beginning or the birth. Usually the term is applied to the genes which one inherits and which determine physical and mental characteristics as the organism develops.

Gynecologist A specialist in medicine who diagnoses and treats diseases of the female tract and reproductive system.

Halsted radical mastectomy The surgical removal of the breast (mastectomy) with incontinuity resection of the axillary lymph nodes and chest wall muscles (pectoralis major and minor muscles).

Hematology The medical science dealing with the study of the blood and blood diseases.

Hematoma A collection of blood that usually occurs outside a blood vessel and may be associated with a leak or injury to that vessel. The collection usually becomes clotted and may become infected. A hematoma may occur in the breast as a lump due to injury and must be watched to be sure that a more serious problem is not present.

Histology Study of the microscopic structure of cells and tissues.

Hormone A chemical substance which is secreted into the body by an endocrine gland (such as ovary or thyroid). It enters the bloodstream and plays a role in regulation of cells and tissues. (Ex. estrogens, progesterone, etc.)

Host resistance The reaction of the cells or tissues of a host (immune response) to a foreign element that may threaten its existence, such as a cancer.

Hot flashes Vague sensations or vasomotor responses with the sensation of heat and sweating that is associated with the menopause.

Hypercoagulability The state of being able to clot or coagulate more easily than normal. The state of hypercoagulability may cause clumping and accumulation of elements that lead to a thrombosis or clot. Hypercoagulability may be necessary for a clumping of cancer cells to form a metastasis.

Hyperplasia A growth of cells causing an excess of cells at a specific anatomical site. (Ex. ductal lining of the breast) This overgrowth may be due to hormonal stimulation, injury or chronic irritation and in the breast is seen at puberty and pregnancy. Hyperplasia is felt by some to be a pre-malignant change in the breast.

Hyperthyroidism An over-activity of the thyroid gland that releases excess thyroid hormones that causes swelling of the gland, nervousness, weight loss, heat loss, tremors, and rapid heart rates.

Hypothyroidism An underactive thyroid gland that does not secrete a normal amount of thyroid hormones. This causes a deficiency state (myxedema) which produces tongue and facial swelling, dry skin, heart enlargement, voice changes, fatigue and usually weight gain. Hypothyroidism can be caused by excessive surgical removal of the gland or disease states which affect its normal function.

Hypogammaglobulinemia Low gammaglobulins (serum protein) in the blood which is a congenital or acquired absence of specific cells.

Hysterectomy The surgical removal of all or part of the uterus.

Immune system A complex system within the host which will resist invasion by a foreign substance (antigen) that may be harmful to the host. This is a form of protection. There is a surveillance system and the ability of the immune system to respond can be favorable or harmful and elicits specific cellular responses.

Immunocytochemistry A chemical and cytological method using monoclonal antibodies to determine if the lymph nodes in the axilla are involved with metastatic tumor or not.

Immunosuppression A suppression of the immune system to respond. This can be normal suppression that is beneficial to the host or it can be self-destructive producing progression of disease (Ex. cancer or infection) and can be artificially induced in some cases by cytotoxic drugs or radiation.

Infiltrating ductal cancer—breast A cancer that originates in the ductal system of the breast and then breaks out of the duct and invades surrounding tissue and produces a firm fibrotic type of tumor.

Informed consent The patient being fully informed or instructed comprehensively about options in treatment in order to select the method that she wants to be used on her.

In situ breast cancer The surface cells show evidence of change indicative of cancer. There is no invasion of the subcutaneous tissue. This is a very low-grade type of breast cancer and there is no evidence of invasion or metastases.

Intraductal papilloma A benign tumor that develops within the ductal system of the breast that has papillary projections. This can cause bleeding and obstruction of the duct and can be single or multiple. It usually is benign but can be malignant.

Inversion of the nipple A turning inward or pulling inward of the nipple of the breast is usually benign or congenital but can be caused by underlying cancer.

Irradiation Treatment of disease with x-ray, radioisotope, ultraviolet, or infrared rays.

Lactation The period of time following childbirth in which the discharge of milk from the breast occurs.

Latissimus dorsi breast reconstruction flap A long muscle on the back and lateral to the breast that is used in musculocutaneous tissue transfer for reconstruction of the breast. The blood supply is kept intact. This type of reconstruction is most often used following radical mastectomy.

Liver scan A radionucleotide scan of the liver. A radioisotope is injected into a vein and concentrates in the liver and then, using a scintillation camera or rectilinear scanner, pictures are taken to detect evidence of cancer spread (metastases). Liver scan is also used as an aid in other diagnoses.

Lobular carcinoma—breast (Infiltrating or invasive) A type of breast cancer that occurs within the terminal ducts and lobules of the breast that is invasive. It is a multicentric type of breast cancer that can be bilateral and is capable of metastases.

Lobular carcinoma in situ—breast A type of cancer that develops in premenopausal breasts in the mammary lobules and does not metastasize (spread). However, it can become invasive in a small percentage of cases.

Local excision—breast Removal of a breast lesion or tumor that is restricted to a local area within the breast. This can be done under local or general anesthesia.

Local recurrence—breast Recurrence of a breast cancer at the local site of excision or of the lumpectomy or mastectomy.

Lymph nodes Encapsulated lymph glands that are connected to the lymphatic system ducts and can be involved with breast cancer spread (metastases). (Ex. lymph glands under the armpit)

Lymphedema of the arm A progressive swelling of the arm due to obstruction within the lymphatic system which can be crippling. Most frequently seen after radical mastectomy and radiation treatment for breast cancer.

Mammography An x-ray technique to define the soft tissues of the breast. A method to produce images of the breast by low voltage x-ray to demonstrate density differences. The image is recorded on x-ray film or selenium coated plates (xeroradiography).

Mastectomy Surgical removal of all breast tissue.
   a) *Simple* Removal of breast tissue only.
   b) *Modified* Removal of all breast tissue and axillary lymph nodes. (glands along the axillary vein and under the armpit)
   c) *Patey type* Removal of all breast tissue and axillary lymph nodes and pectoralis minor muscle.
   d) *Radical* Removal of all breast tissue, including chest wall muscles (pectoralis major and minor muscles) and axillary lymph nodes.

Menopause The time in the lifespan of a female when the menstrual cycle ends. Usually between the ages of 40–55. Ovarian function is reduced and estrogen secretion decreases or stops. A surgical menopause is due to surgical removal of the uterus and ovaries.

Metabolism The physical and chemical process by which a living organism grows, maintains its nutrition, and produces energy and its capability to reproduce.

Metastasis To form a new focus of a disease such as cancer by distant spread from its primary site. This usually occurs through lymphatic channels or blood vessels.

Micrometastases The spread of cancer that can only be seen under a microscope.

Minimal cancer Minimal cancers of the breast are nonpalpable tumors detected by mammography that measure less than 5mm. in diameter. (Ex. lobular cancer in situ, intraductal cancer)

Mittelschmerz Pelvic pain that occurs in the middle of the menstrual cycle at the time of ovulation.

Monoclonal antibodies Specific antibodies derived from a single cell (cloning) which can be used to fight diseases such as cancer.

Monocyte The largest type of white blood cell, formed in the bone marrow, and capable of ingesting bacteria, viruses and tissue debris.

Morbidity rate The number of cases per year of a specific disease per 100,000 people. Sick rate.

Morphology The study of the form and structure of an organism, organ, or its parts including tissues and cells.

Multicentric breast cancer The development of cancer in multiple and separate areas of the breast.

Myriad An indefinite, immense number.

Necrosis The death and breakdown of tissues which are surrounded by healthy tissues.

Needle localization—breast A thin wire is introduced into the breast under x-ray control to pinpoint suspected minimal breast cancers. (Local anesthesia is usually used)

Neovascularization The development of blood vessels associated with tumor growth in which the lining (endothelium) of the blood vessels proliferate.

Nephrotoxic A substance such as a chemical or chemotherapeutic agent that is toxic or damaging to the structure and function of the kidneys. This damage can progress on to renal failure.

Neuroendocrine system The interaction that occurs between the nervous system and the endocrine system. An example is the hypothalamic (brain), pituitary, and adrenal gland and their effects that occur with stress.

Nuclear magnetic resonance (NMR) An imaging technique that uses a magnet and electrical coil to transmit radio waves through the body to form a cross-sectional picture.

Nucleus A spheroidal body within the cell that is separate from the cytoplasm that contains the chromosomes and is the site of DNA repliation.

Obstetrician A physician that primarily deals with the diagnosis and management of pregnancy, labor and the post-partum care of the female.

Occult cancer An obscure or hidden cancer in which the primary site can not be determined.

Omentum A fold of the lining of the abdomen containing thick fatty fibrous tissue that extends from the stomach to adjacent organs in the abdomen. (an apron type of covering over the abdominal organs)

Oncogenes Tumor genes that are present in the body that can be activated by cancer agents such as radiation or chemicals that can cause cells to become cancer.

Oncologist A physician whose specialty is the diagnosis and treatment of tumors. Most oncologists have had additional specialized training in a major cancer center.

Ophorectomy The surgical removal of an ovary or ovaries.

Osteoporosis A condition that most commonly affects females after the menopause in which there is a washing out or demineralization of bone that can cause pain and deformity of the spine and pathological fractures (breaks) can develop.

Ovaries Two reproductive glands in the female, containing the ova or germ cells.

Paget's Disease of the nipple A ductal cancer of the breast that involves the skin of the nipple and areola. A crusting, scaly, red dermatitis type of lesion.

Palpation Examination by feeling with the hand.

Pathology The branch of medicine which deals with the changes in the body produced by disease.

Pectoralis muscles Pectoralis major and minor muscles directly under the breast and attached to the chest wall. The muscles removed in a radical mastectomy.

Pelvic inflammatory disease (PID) An acute or chronic inflammatory disease of the pelvic organs which occurs predominately in young sexually active females and can lead to infertility.

Pesticides Poisons used to destroy pests that inhibit the growth of plants or animals. (Ex. insecticides, fungicides, rodenticides)

Pleomorphism The unusual, irregular, and abnormal cell and nuclear shapes that occur in various distinct forms of the cancer cell.

Pleural effusion The collection of fluid between the serous membrane that covers the lungs (visceral pleura) and the lining of the chest (parental pleura) cavity (thorax).

Progesterone A female sex hormone secreted by the ovaries that prepares the uterus for pregnancy and the breasts for lactation.

Progestin is the synthetic form of progesterone.

Progestogen is a substance prossessing progestational activity also used in oral contraceptives.

Prolactin A hormone in the pituitary gland that stimulates lactation and the production of progesterone by the ovaries. Measured by radioimmune assay technique.

Prophylactic castration The removal of the ovaries in patients with breast cancer to, hopefully, prevent metastases. Also used in the treatment of breast cancer after spread has occurred.

Prophylactic subcutaneous mastectomy Removing all of the breast tissue subcutaneously as a preventative measure for breast cancer. (This is a misnomer since it is almost impossible to remove all breast tissue with this operation)

Prosthetic device A device that serves as a substitute such as a silicone gel plastic bag to replace the mound of the breast after mastectomy.

Radiation A stream of particles emitted by a radioactive material. This can be used for diagnostic purposes or treatment and the biological effects can be both helpful and harmful.

Radioisotope An isotope which is radioactive. Injection of isotopes which concentrate in the bones or liver are used to detect spread of breast cancer (metastases to that site).

Red blood cells Red blood cells are formed in the bone marrow. Their main function is oxygen transport and they survive for approximately 120 days in the circulation.

Regional metastases Spread of a primary cancer to a regional site, such as breast cancer spreading to the lymph nodes under the armpit.

Rehabilitation Restoring a person to healthy, useful activity following surgery such as mastectomy.

Replacement hormone therapy The use of hormones such as estrogen to replace the natural hormones lost when an oophorectomy (ovaries) and hysterectomy (uterus) is done.

Scintillation camera Device used to magnify radiation and record the results for the diagnosis of cancer or other disorders.

Scirrhous cancer—breast A cancer of the breast with a hard, firm, fibrous consistency, usually an infiltrating ductal carcinoma, that can be confused with other diagnoses.

Screening mammography A female over a specified age (40 yrs.) has a mammography done as a routine procedure, usually once a year, to see if the breast is involved with cancer.

Silicone Synthetic compound used in breast implants because of its flexibility, resilience and tensile strength. Usually a gel inside a plastic bag.

Skin dimpling The indentation of the skin, which can be seen, that indicates the possibility of a cancer in the breast. Usually due to ligaments just under the skin surface that are involved with cancer and are attached to the skin.

Slough A mass or layer of dead tissue which separates from the surrounding or underlying living tissue.

Stage of breast disease A method of staging breast cancer based on the size of the tumor, whether regional axillary lymph nodes are involved, whether the skin, chest muscles, distant lymph nodes or blood stream spread has occurred.

Systemic disease As related to breast disease, means that the primary tumor has disseminated and spread to distal sites, such as the liver, chest, brain, bones, or soft tissues.

Tamoxifen An estrogen blocking agent (drug) used in the preventative and prophylactic treatment of breast cancer.

Thermography A method of measuring temperature variations in the breast that may contain cancer. Breast tumors show up as "hot spots" on the thermogram.

Thrombin An enzyme which is necessary for blood to clot.

Thrombophlebitis A clot that usually forms in a vein and causes an inflammatory response. The clot is usually due to stasis or pooling of blood and occurs most often in the lower extremities and pelvis.

Thyroid gland Gland located in the lower neck that plays a large role in metabolic functions. The gland can become enlarged due to stress or hyper or hypo functioning. Normal iodine intake is necessary for normal function.

Triglycerides Form in which dietary fat is stored in the body, consisting of glycerol combined with three fatty-acid molecules.

Tummy tuck—breast reconstruction Resection of the lower skin of the abdomen with the blood supply (rectus muscles) transplanted to the chest wall and breast area and used for breast reconstruction and abdominal cosmesis.

Ultrasonography (ultrasound) A method in which high frequency sound waves are used to outline anatomical structures of the body. High frequency sounds are transmitted through the body and the echoes are detected and displayed on a television screen. It is used primarily to determine if a structure is solid or liquid and is useful in detecting breast cysts in young females with firm fibrous breasts. (No radiation effect occurs)

Uterus The womb or hollow muscular organ lined by epithelium in the pelvis that receives and holds the fertilized egg, feeds and nourishes the developing embryo and fetus. Removed during hysterectomy.

Vaginitis—atrophic An inflammation of the vagina that occurs after menopause in which the vaginal tissue becomes thin and dry due to decreased estrogen production.

White blood cells The cells in blood that remain after the red cells have been removed. The white cells play a role in defense against infection and T cell lymphocytes and B cell lymphocytes (a part of the total number of white cells) play a role in the immune system against cancer.

Xeroradiography X-ray imaging technique in which images of breast tissue are reproduced on a xerox plate rather than on conventional x-ray film.

References

1. Wilson, R. E., M.D., Donegan, W.L., M.D., Mettlin, Curtis, Ph.D., Nachimuthu, Natarjan, M.D., Stuart, Charles, R., Murphy, Gerald P. The 1982 National Survey of the Breast in the United States by the American College of Surgeons. Surg. Gyn., Obst. Vol. 159, No. 4 October, 1984 p. 309–317.
2. Axtell, L.M., Asire, A.J., Myers, M.D. (eds): Cancer patient survival. Rep No. 5, DHEW Pub. No. (NIH) 77–992. Bethesda, National Cancer Institute, 1976.
3. Lilienfeld, Abraham M. The epidemiology of breast cancer. Cancer Res. 1963, 23:1503.
4. Macklin, Madge T. Comparison of the number of breast cancer deaths observed in relatives of breast cancer patients, and the number expected on the basis of mortality rates. J. Nat'l. Cancer Inst., 1959, 22:927.
5. Fraumeni, J.F., Jr., Lloyd, J.W., Smith, E.M., and Wagoner, J.K. Cancer mortality among nuns: role of marital status in etiology of neoplastic disease in women. J. Nat'l. Cancer Inst. 1969, 42:455.
6. Trichopoulos, D., MacMahon, B., and Cole, P. Menopause and breast cancer risk. J. Nat'l. Cancer Inst. 1972, 48:605.
7. Finley, J.W. and Bogardus, G.M. Breast cancer and thyroid disease. Quart. Rev. Surg. 1960, 17:139–147
8. Stadel, B.V. Dietary iodine and risk of breast, endometrial, and ovarian cancer. Lancet 1976, 1:890–891.
9. Backwinkel, L. and Jackson, A.S. Some features of breast cancer and thyroid deficiency—report of 280 cases. Cancer. 1964, 17:1174–1176.
10. Graham, S., Levin, M., and Lilienfeld, A. The socio-economic distri-

bution of cancer in various sites in Buffalo, NY 1948–1952. Cancer. 1960, 13:180–191.

11. Gallup, Omnibus. A survey concerning cigarette smoking, health check-ups, cancer detection tests. A summary of the findings. Conducted for: the American Cancer Society Inc. The Gallup Organization Inc., GO 7695 T, January, 1977.

12. Mahoney, L.J., Bird, B.L., Cooke, G.M. Annual clinical examination: the best available screening test for breast cancer. N. Engl. J. Med. 1979 301:315–316.

13. Humphrey, Loren J. Multidisciplinary cancer care. Oncology Times, May, 1983, Vol. V, No. 5.

14. Martin, Hayes E., and Ellis, Edward B. Biopsy by needle puncture and aspiration. Ann. Surg. 1930, 32:169.

15. Saphir, Otto. Early diagnosis of breast lesions. J.A.M.A., 1952, Vol. 150, No. 9, 859–861.

16. Robbins, G.F., Brothers, J.H., III, Eberhart, W.F. and Quan, S. Is as-piration biopsy of breast cancer dangerous to patients? Cancer, 1974, 7:774–778.

17. Berg, John W., and Robbins, G.F. A late look at the safety of aspiration biopsy. Cancer, 1962, 15:826–7.

18. Vorherr, H. Study indicates that multihole needle may be more accurate for breast aspiration biopsy. Oncology Times, Dec. 1983, Vol. V, #12, p. 4.

19. Kreuzer, G. and Zajicek, J. Cytologic diagnosis of mammary tumors from aspiration biopsy smears III studies on 200 carcinomas with false negative or doubtful cytologic reports. Acta Cytol 1972, 16:249.

20. Ruzicka, Francis F., Jr., Kaufman, Leonard, Shapiro, Gerald, Perez, Joseph V., and Grossi, Carlo, E. Xeromammography and film mammography—A comparative study. Radiology, 1965, 85:260–269.

21. Wolfe, John N. Xerography of the breast. Radiology, 1968. 91:231–240.

22. Martin, John E. and Gallager, H. Stephen. Mammographic diagnosis of minimal breast cancer. Cancer, 1971, 28:1519–1526.

23. Frankl, Gloria and Rosenfeld, David D. Xeroradiographic detection of occult breast cancer. Cancer, 1975, 35:542–548.

24. Gautherie, Michel, Gross, Charles M. Breast thermography and cancer risk prediction. Cancer, 1980. 45:51–56.

25. Stark, A.M. and Way, S. The screening of well women for the early detection of breast cancer using clinical examinations with thermography and mammography. Cancer, 1974, 33:1671–1679.

26. Wallace, J.D. and Dodd, G.D. Thermography in the diagnosis of breast cancer. Radiology, 1968, 91:679–685.

27. Black, F. (1946) Physical Review. 70:460–474.

28. Purcell, E.M., Torrey, H.C., Pound, R.V. (1946) Physical Review 69:37–38.

29. Doyle, F.H., Gore, J.C., Perrnock, J.M. et al. 1981, Lancet 53, 57.

30. Wells, C.A., Heryet, A., Brochier, J., Gatter, K.C., and Mason, D.Y. The immunocytochemical detection of axillary micrometastases in breast cancer. Br. J. Cancer, 1984, 50:193–197.

31. Friedman, Nathan B. Pathologist warns radiation therapy not conservative, hits healthy tissue. Hospital Tribune Report, July 18, 1984, p. 18.

32. Mettler, Fred A., Jr., Hempelmann, Louis H., Dutton, Arthur M., Pifer, James, W., Toyooka, Edward T., Ames, Wendell R. Breast neoplasms in women treated with x-rays for acute postpartum mastitis. A pilot study. J. Nat'l. Cancer Inst., 1969, 43:803–811.

33. Dvoretsky, Philip M., Woodard, Elizabeth, Bonfiglio, Thomas A., Hempelmann, Louis H., and Morse, Ilka P. The pathology of breast cancer in women irradiated for acute postpartum mastitis. Cancer, 1980, 46:2257–2262.

34. Mackenzie, I. Breast cancer following multiple fluoroscopies. Br. J. Ca., 1965, 19:1–8.

35. Wanebo, C.K., Johnson, K.G., Sato, K., and Thorslund, T.W. Breast cancer after exposure to the atomic bombings of Hiroshima and Nagasaki. N.E. J. Med. 1968, Vol. 279, No. 13, 667–671.

36. Beir Report. Advisory Committee on the Biological Effects of ionizing radiations, National Academy of Sciences—National Research Council: The effects on populations of exposure to low levels of ionizing radiation. U.S. Gov't. Print. Off., Washington, D.C., 1972.

37. Harvey, E.B., Boice, J.D., Jr., Honeyman, M., Flannery, J.T. Prenatal x-ray exposure and childhood cancer in twins. N.E. J. Med. 1985, 312:541–545.

38. Hutchinson, W.B., Thomas, D.B., Hamlin, W.B., Roth, G.J., Peterson, A.V., Williams, B. Risk of breast cancer in women with benign breast disease. JNCI July, 1980, Vol. 65, No. 1, 13–20.

39. Soini, I., Aine, R., Lauslahti, K., Hakama, M. Independent risk factors of benign and malignant breast lesions. Amer. J. Epidemiology, 1981, Vol. 114, No. 4, 507–512.

40. Kodijn, D., Winger, E.E., Morgenstern, N.L., Chen, U. Chronic mastopathy and breast cancer. A follow-up study. Cancer, 1977, 39:2603–2607.

41. Barber, H.R.K., Braber, E.A. *Surgical disease in pregnancy*. Philadelphia, W.B. Saunders Company, 1974, 303–309, 728–729.

42. Dilman, V.M. Metabolic immunodepression which increases the risk of cancer. Lancet, Dec. 10, 1977, 1207–1209.

43. White, T.T. Carcinoma of the breast in the pregnant and the nursing patient. Review of 1375 cases. Am. J. Obstet. Gynec. 1955, 69:1277–1286.

44. Jones, R., Wernerman, B. MOOP (nitrogen mustard, vincristine, procarbazine, and prednisone) given during pregnancy. Obstet. Gynecol. 1979, 54:477–478.

45. Geggie, Peter H.S. Breast cancer in pregnant women. C.M.A. Journal, Sept. 1, 1982, 127:358–359.

46. MacMahon, B., Lin, T.M., Lowe, C.R. et al. Lactation and cancer of the breast, a summary of an international study. Bull. W.H.O. 1970, 42:185–194.

47. Lee, T.N., Horz, J.M. Significance of ovarian metastases in therapeutic oophorectomy for advanced breast cancer. Cancer, 1971, 27:1374–1378.

48. Kennedy, B.J., Mielke, P.W., Fortuny, I.E. Therapeutic abortion versus prophylactic castration in mammary carcinoma. Surg. Gynec. Obstet. 1964, 118:524–540.

49. Greenberg, E.R., Barnes, A.B., Resseguie, L., Barrett, J.A., Burnside, S., Lanza, L.L., Neff, R.K., Stevens, M., Young, R.H., Colton, T. Breast cancer in mothers given Diethylstilbestrol in pregnancy. N. Eng. J. Med. 1984, 311:1393–8.

50. Peters, M.V. The effect of pregnancy in breast cancer in: Prognostic factors in breast cancer. Edited by A.P.M. Forest and P.B. Kunkler, London: E. & S. Livingstone 1968, pp. 65–80.

51. Harvey, J.C., Rosen, P.P., Ashikari, R., Robbins, G.F., Kinne, D.W. The effect of pregnancy on the prognosis of carcinoma of the breast following radical mastectomy. Surg. Gynecol. Obstet. 1981, 153:723–725.

52. Ross, R.K., Paganini-Hill, A., Gerkins, V.R., Mack, T.M., Pfeffer, R., Arthur, M., Henderson, B.E. A case control study of menopause estrogen therapy and breast cancer. JAMA 1980, 243:1635–1639.

53. Cutler, S.J., Young, J.L. (eds.) *Third National Cancer Survey Incidence Data* National Cancer Institute Monograph 41. Government Printing Office, 1975.

54. Lucas, W.E. Causal relationships between endocrine-metabolic variables in patients with endometrial carcinoma. Obstet-Gynecol. Survey 1974, 29:507.

55. Cutts, J.H., Nobel, R.L. Estrone-induced mammary tumors in the rat. Cancer Res. 1964, 24:1116–1123.

56. Antunes, C.M.F., Stolley, P.D., Rosenshein, M.B. et al. Endometrial cancer and estrogen use. Report of a large case control study. N.Eng. J. Med. 1979, 300:9.

57. Gray, L.A., Jr., Christopherson, W.M., Hoover, R. Estrogens and endometrial cancer. Obstet. Gynecol. 1977, 49:385.

58. Jelovk, F.R., Hammond, C.B., Woodward, B.H. et al. Risks of exogenous estrogen therapy and endometrial cancer. Am. J. Obstet. Gynecol. 1980, 137:85.

59. Jick, H., Watkins, R.N., Hunter, J.R. et al. Replacement estrogens and endometrial cancer. N. Eng. J. Med. 1979, 300:218.

60. Pike, M.C., Henderson, B.E., Krailo, M.D., Duke, A. Breast cancer in young women and use of oral contraceptives: Possible modifying effect of formulation and age at use. Lancet, 1983, II:926.

61. Lincoln, R. The pill, breast and cervical cancer and the role of progestogen in arterial disease. Family Planning Perspectives. March–April 1984, Vol. 16, No. 2.

62. Ferguson, D.J.P., Anderson, T.J. Morphological evaluation of cell turnover in relation to the menstrual cycle in the resting human breast. British J. of Cancer 1981, 44:177.

63. Grattarola, R. Anovulation and increased androgenic activity as breast cancer risk in women with fibrocystic disease of the breast. Cancer Res. 1978, 38:3051–4.

64. MacMahon, B., Cole, P., Lin, T.M. et al. Age at first birth and breast cancer risk. Bull. W.H.O. 1970, 43:209–21.

65. Drife, J.O. Breast cancer, pregnancy and the pill. British Med. J., Sept. 19, 1981, 283:778–779.

66. Brinton, L.A., Vessey, M.P., Flavel, R. et al. Risk factors for benign breast disease. Amer. J. Epidemiol. 1981, 113(3)203–14.

67. Greenspon, A.R., Hatcher, R.A., Moore, M. et al. The association of depomedroxyprogesterone acetate and breast caner. Contraception 1980, 21(6):563–9.

68. Halsted, W.S. The treatment of wounds with especial reference to the value of the blood clot in the management of dead spaces. Johns Hopkins Hospital Reports, 1891, 2:255–316.

69. Roentgen, W.C. On a new kind of rays. Clinical Orthopaedics and related research (J.B. Lippincott Co.) 1969, 65:3–8.

70. Kraft, E., Finby, N. Wilhelm Conrad Roentgen (1845–1923) Discoverer of x-ray. 1974, 74:2066–70.

71. McWhirter, R. Simple mastectomy and radiotherapy in the treatment of breast cancer. Brit. J. Radiol. March 1955, 28:128–139.

72. Stewart, H.J. and Sutherland, I. World J. Surg., 1976.

73. Stewart, H.J. Controlled trials in the treatment of "early" breast cancer: a review of published results. World J. Surg. 1977, 1:309–313.

74. Bonadonna, G., Brusamolino, E., Valagussa, P., Rossi, A., Brugnatelli, L., Brambilla, C., DeLena, M., Tancini, G., Bajetta, E., Musumeci, R., Veronesi, U. Combination chemotherapy as an adjuvant treatment in operable breast cancer. N. Eng. J. Med. 1976, 294:405–410.

75. Peters, M.V. Wedge resection and irradiation—an effective treatment in early breast cancer. JAMA, 1967, 200:144–145.

76. Meyer, K.K., Weaver, D.R., Luft, W.C., Boselli, B.D. Lymphocyte

immune deficiency following irradiation for carcinoma of the breast. Front. Radiation Ther. Onc. 1972, 7, 179, edit. J.M. Vaeth. S. Karger, Basel.

77. Slater, J.M., Ngo, E. and Lau, B.H.S. Effect of therapeutic irradiation on the immune responses. Amer. J. Roentgenol. 1976, 126, 313.

78. Fisher, B., Bauer, M., Margolese, R., Poisson, R., Pilch, Y., Redmond, C., Fisher, E., Wolmark, N., Deutsch, M., Montague, E., Saffer, E., Wickerham, L., Lernes, H., Glass, A., Shibata, H., Deckers, P., Ketcham, A., Oishi, R., Russell, I. Five-Year results of a randomized clinical trial comparing total mastectomy and segmental mastectomy with or without radiation in the treatment of breast cancer. N. Eng. J. Med. March 14, 1985, 312:665–673.

79. Davis, J.B. Carcinoma of the breast. Arch. Surg. 1957, 74:758–769.

80. Farrow, J.H., Fracchia, A.A., Robbins, G.F., Castro, E. Simple excision or biopsy plus radiation therapy as the primary treatment for potentially curable cancer of the breast. Cancer, 1971, 28:1195–1201.

81. Pigott, J., Nichols, R., Maddox, W.A., Balch, C.M. (Univ. of Alabama Med. Center, Birmingham) Surg. Gynecol. Obstet. March 1984, 158:255–259.

82. Gallagher, H.S., Martin, J.E. Early phases in the development of breast cancer. Cancer, 1969, 24:1170–1178.

83. Rosen, P.P., Fracchia, A.A., Urban, J.A. Schottenfeld, D., Robbins, G.F. Residual mammary carcinoma following simulated partial mastectomy. Cancer 1975, 35:739–47.

84. Lesser, M.L., Rosen, P.P., Kinne, D.W. Multicentricity and bilaterality in invasive breast carcinoma. Surgery 1982, 91:234–240.

85. Peters, M.V. Wedge resection and irradiation—an effective treatment in early breast cancer. JAMA, 1967, 200:144–145.

86. MacMahan, B., Cole, P., Brown, J. Etiology of human breast cancer: A review, 1973, J. Nat'l Cancer Inst. 50:21–42.

87. Armstrong, B., Doll, R. Environmental factors and cancer incidence and mortality in different countries with special reference to dietary practices. Int. J. Cancer 1975, 15:617–631.

88. Hirayanna, T. Changing pattern of cancer in Japan with special reference to the decrease in stomach cancer mortality. H.H. Hiatt, 1977, pp. 55–75.

89. Watson, J.D., Winsten, J.A. eds. *Origins of human cancer, Book A. Incidence of cancer in humans.* Cold Spring Harbor Laboratory, Cold Spring Harbor, N.Y.

90. Dunn, J.E., Jr. Breast cancer among American Japanese in the San Francisco Bay area. Nat'l Cancer Inst. Monogr. 1977, 47:157–160.

91. *Diet, Nutrition and Cancer,* National Academy Press, 1982.

92. Pauling, L. Vitamin C therapy of advanced cancer. N. Engl. J. Med., 1980, 302:694.

93. Cameron, E., Pauling L. Supplemental ascorbate in the supportive treatment of cancer; prolongation of survival times in terminal human cancer. Proc. Nat'l Acad. Sci. U.S.A. 1976, 73:3685–9.

94. Moertel, C.G., Feming, T.R., Creagan, E.T., Rubin, J., O'Connell, M.J., Awes, M.M. High dose vitamin C versus placebo in the treatment of patients with advanced cancer who have had no prior chemotherapy. N. Eng. J. Med. 1985, 312–137–41.

95. Minton, J.P., Foecking, M.K., Webster, D.J.T., Matthews, R.H. Caffeine, cyclic nucleotides, and breast disease. Surgery, 1979, 86:105.

96. Minton, J.P., Foecking, M.K., Webster, D.J.T., Matthews, R.H. Response of fibrocystic disease to caffeine withdrawal and correlation of cyclic nucleotides with breast disease. Am. Obstet. Gynec. 1979, 135:157.

97. Rosenberg, L., Slone, D., Shapiro, S. Breast cancer and alcohol beverage consumption. Lancet 1982, i:267–71.

98. Begy, C.B., Walker, A.M., Wessen, B., Zelen, M. Alcohol consumption and breast cancer. Lancet 1983, i:293–94.

99. World Health Organization 1964 cancer agents that surround us. World Health 1964, (Sep.):16–17.

100. Corrigan, J.J., Jr. and Marcus, F.I. Coagulopathy associated with vitamin E ingestion. J.A.M.A. 1974, 230:1300.

101. Corrigan, J.J., Jr. and Ulfers, L.L. Effect of vitamin E on prothrombin levels in a warfarin induced vitamin K deficiency. Amer. J. Clin. Nutr. 1981, 34:1701.

102. Selye, H. A syndrome produced by diverse nocuous agents. Nature (Lond.) 1936, 138:32.

103. Paget, J. *Surgical Pathology, 2nd ed.* Longmans Green, London, 1870, p. 800.

104. Guy R. *An Essay on Scirrhous Tumours and Cancers.* Churchill, London (1759). Cited in Goldfarb D., Driesen, J., and Cole, D. Psychophysiologic aspects of malignancy. Am. J. Psychiat. 123, 1545 (1967).

105. Paget, S. The distribution of secondary growths in cancer of the breast. The Lancet. 1889, pp. 571–73.

106. Cole, W.H. Spontaneous regression of cancer. The metabolic triumph of the host. Ann. N.Y. Acad. Sci. 1974, 250:111–141.

107. Keller, S.E., Ioachim, H.L., Pearse, T., Siletti, D.M. Decreased T-lymphocytes in patients with mammary cancer. Amer. J. Clin. Path. 1976, 65:445–449.

108. Cheema, A.R., Hersh, E.M. Patient survival after chemotherapy and its relationship to in vitro lymphocyte blastogenesis. Cancer 1971, 28:851–855.

109. Dilman, V.M. Metabolic immunodepression which increases the risk of cancer. Lancet, Dec. 10, 1977, 1207–1209.

110. Mertin, J., Hunt, R. *Proc. Natn. Acad. Sci.* 1976, 73:928.
111. Temin, H.M., *J Cell. Comp. Physiol.* 1969, 74:9.
112. Dilman, V.M., Bobrov, Ju. F. Sovremennze Problemi Oncologil; p.76. Leningrad, 1966.
113. Stjernsward, J., Jondal, M., Vanky, F., Wigzell, H., Sealy, R. Lymphopenia and change in distribution of human B & T lymphocytes in peripheral blood induced by irradiation for mammary cancer. Lancet, 1972, I:1352–1356.
114. Hoover, R., Fraumeni, J.F., Jr. Risk of cancer in renal transplant recipients. Lancet, 1973, 2:55–57.
115. Penn, I. Second malignant neoplasms associated with immunosuppressive medications. Cancer 1976, 37:1024–1032.
116. Rollin, Betty, *First You Cry.* Signet, New York, 1977.
117. Deck, K.B., Kern, W.H. Local recurrence of breast cancer. Arch. Surg. 1976, 111:323–325.
118. Shah, J.P., Urban, J.A. Full thickness chest wall resection for recurrent breast carcinoma involving the bony chest wall. Cancer, 1975, 35:567–573.
119. Fisher, B., Ravdin, R.G., Ausman, R.K., Slack, N.H., Moore, G.E., Noer, R.J. Surgical adjuvant chemotherapy in cancer of the breast: results of a decade of cooperative investigation. Annals of Surgery 1968, 168:337.
120. Cronin, T., Gerow, F.J. Augmentation mammoplasty; a new natural feel prosthesis in transactions of the third International Congress of Plastic Surgery. Excerpta Medica Foundation, Amsterdam, 1963.
121. Snyderman, R.K., Guthrie, R.H. Reconstruction of the female breast following radical mastectomy. Plastic and Reconstructive Surgery 1971, 47(6):565–567.
122. d'Este, S., La technique de L'amputation de La mammelle pour carcinome mammairre. Rev. Chir. 1912, 45:164.
123. Davis, H.H., Tollman, P., Brush, J.H. Huge chondrosarcoma of rib. Report of a case. Surgery, 1949, 26:699.
124. Orticochea, M. The musculo-cutaneous flap method: an immediate and heroic substitute for the method of delay. Br. J. Plastic Surg. 1972, 25:106.
125. Radovan, C. Breast reconstruction after mastectomy using the temporary expander. Plas. Reconstr. Surgery 1982, 69:195.
126. Becker, H. Breast reconstruction using an inflatable breast implant with detachable reservoir. Plastic and Reconstr. Surg. 1984, 73(4):678–683.
127. Arnold, P.G., Hartrampf, C.R., Jurkiewicz, M.J. One stage reconstruction of the breast using the transposed greater omentum. Plast. & Reconstr. Surg. 1976, 57:520–522.
128, Robbins, T.H. Rectus abdominis myocutaneous flap for breast reconstruction. Aust. N.Z. J. Surg. 1979, 49:527.

129. Dinner, M.I., Labandter, H.P., Dowden, R.V. The role of the rectus abdominis myocutaneous flap in breast reconstruction. Plastic Reconstr. Surg. 1982, 69(2):209.

130. Rose, J.H., Jr. Carcinoma in a transplanted nipple. Arch. Surg. 1980, 115:1131–1132.

131. Cucin, R.L., Gastos, J.P. Implantation of breast cancer in a transplanted nipple: a plea for pre-operative screening. Ca A Cancer Journal for Clinicians. 1981, 31(5):281–283.

132. Bartlett, W. An anatomical substitute for the female breast. Ann Surg. 1917, 66:208.

133. Simonton, O.C. *Getting Well Again,* J.P. Tarcher, Los Angeles, 1978.

134. Kuehn, P.G. Quality of survival of the cancer patient, Hartford Unit, American Cancer Society publication, 1969.

135. Priestman, T.J., Bavin, M. Evaluation of quality of life in patients receiving treatment for advanced breast cancer. Lancet, 1976, 1:899–901.

136. Priestman, T.J. Quality of life after cytotoxic chemotherapy. J. Royal Soc. Med. 1984, 77:492–495.

137. American Cancer Society, 1985, Cancer Facts & Figures.

138. Sappey, P.C. Anatomie, Physiologie, Pathologie des Vaisseauz Lymphatique Consideres chez l'Homme et les Vertebris. Paris, A. Delahaye and E. Lecrosnie 18, [74] 85.

139. Rouviere, H. Anatomie des Lymphatiques de L'homme Paris, Masson, et cie, 1932, 197–240.

140. Rotter, J. Zur Topographie des mamma-carcinomas. Arch Klin Chir, 1899, 58:346.

141. Handley, R.S. The surgical anatomy of the breast. Baltimore, 1955, The Williams and Wilkern Co. 2:28–52.

142. Virchow, R. Gesammelte Abhandlungen Zur Wissenschaftlichen Medicin Frankfort A.M., 1856. Von Meidlinger Sohn u Comp.

143. Trousseau, A. Clinique Medicale de L'Hotel—Dieu de Paris, 1868, 3:35. J.B. Balliere et fils.

144. Wood, Sumner, Jr., Yardley, John H., Holyoke, E. Douglas. The relationship between intravascular coagulation and the formation of pulmonary metastases in mice injected intravenously with tumor suspension. Proceedings of the American Assoc. for Cancer Research, 1957, 2:260.

145. Song, J., From, P., Morrissey, W.J., Sams, J. Circulating cancer cells; Pre- and post-chemotherapy observations. Cancer, 1971, 28:553.

146. Paget, Stephen, The distribution of secondary growths in cancer of the breast. The Lancet. 1889, pp. 571–73.

147. Fuchs. Sarkom des Uvealtractus, 1882.

148. Kuehn, Paul G., Beckett, Ronald, Reed, John F. Tissue specificity in

multiple primary malignancies (A study of 460 cases). American Journal of Surgery, Feb. 1966, Vol. 111, No. 2, 164–167.

149. Genital wart virus infections: nuisance or potentially lethal? British Medical Journal 1984, 288:No. 6419, pp. 735–737.

150. Goldsmith, Marsha F. Papillomavirus invades esophagus, incidence seems to be increasing. JAMA, 1984, 251:No. 17, pp. 2185–2187.

ABOUT THE AUTHOR

PAUL KUEHN is a Surgical Oncologist, a graduate of Trinity College and the University of Rochester Medical School. He completed a general surgical residency at Hartford Hospital and then received a National Cancer Institute Fellowship for further studies in cancer at the Memorial Sloan Kettering Cancer Center in New York City where he was a senior resident in Surgical Oncology.

He was the Chairman of the American Cancer Society's National award winning program titled Quality of Survival of the Cancer Patient. He is a past President of the Hartford Unit of the American Cancer Society and of the Connecticut Division of the American Cancer Society and has also served as Chairman of the Cancer Commission for New England for the American College of Surgeons.

He is currently President of the New England Cancer Society.

The author of numerous articles on cancer for national medical journals, he is recognized as one of our country's leading cancer specialists.